The Matrix & The Forbidden Knowledge

Part 5 - Finale

By Malik Bade

@ACENSIONRISE

Tables of Content

Chapter 17: The Spirit World

Chapter 17: The Spirit World

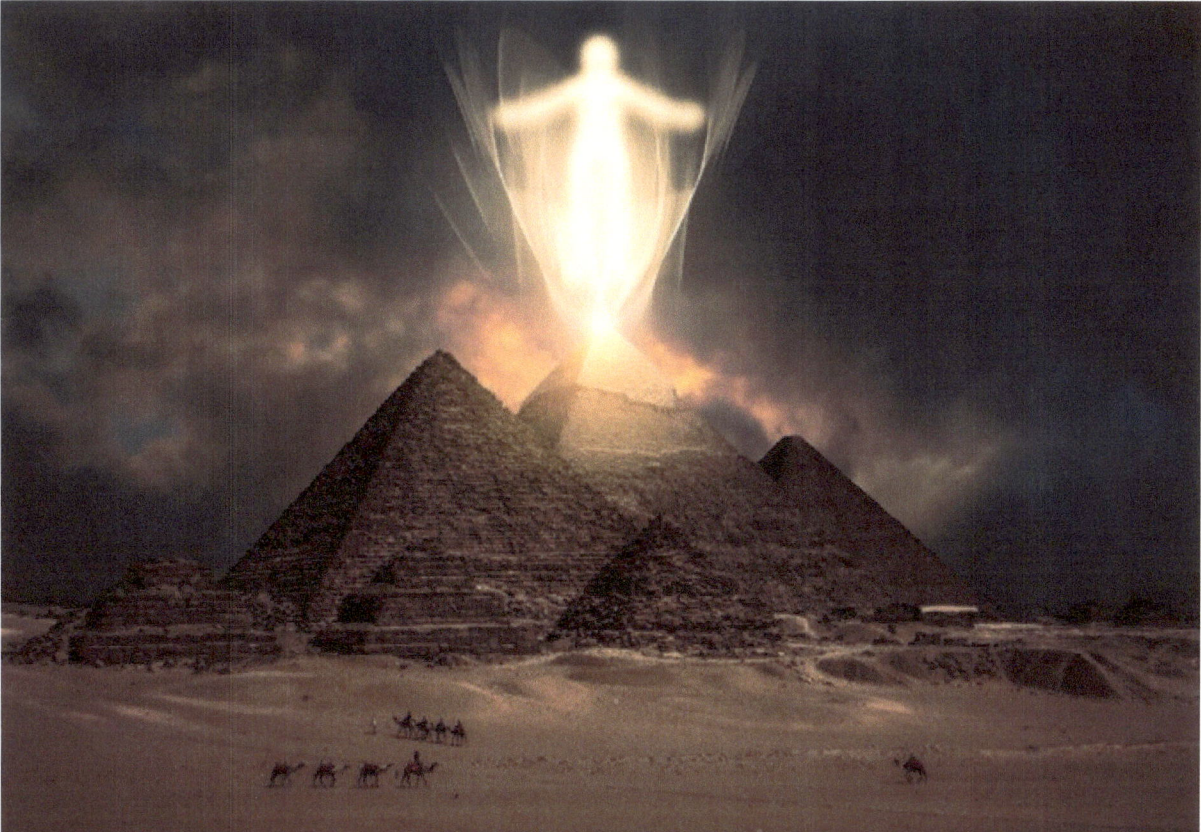

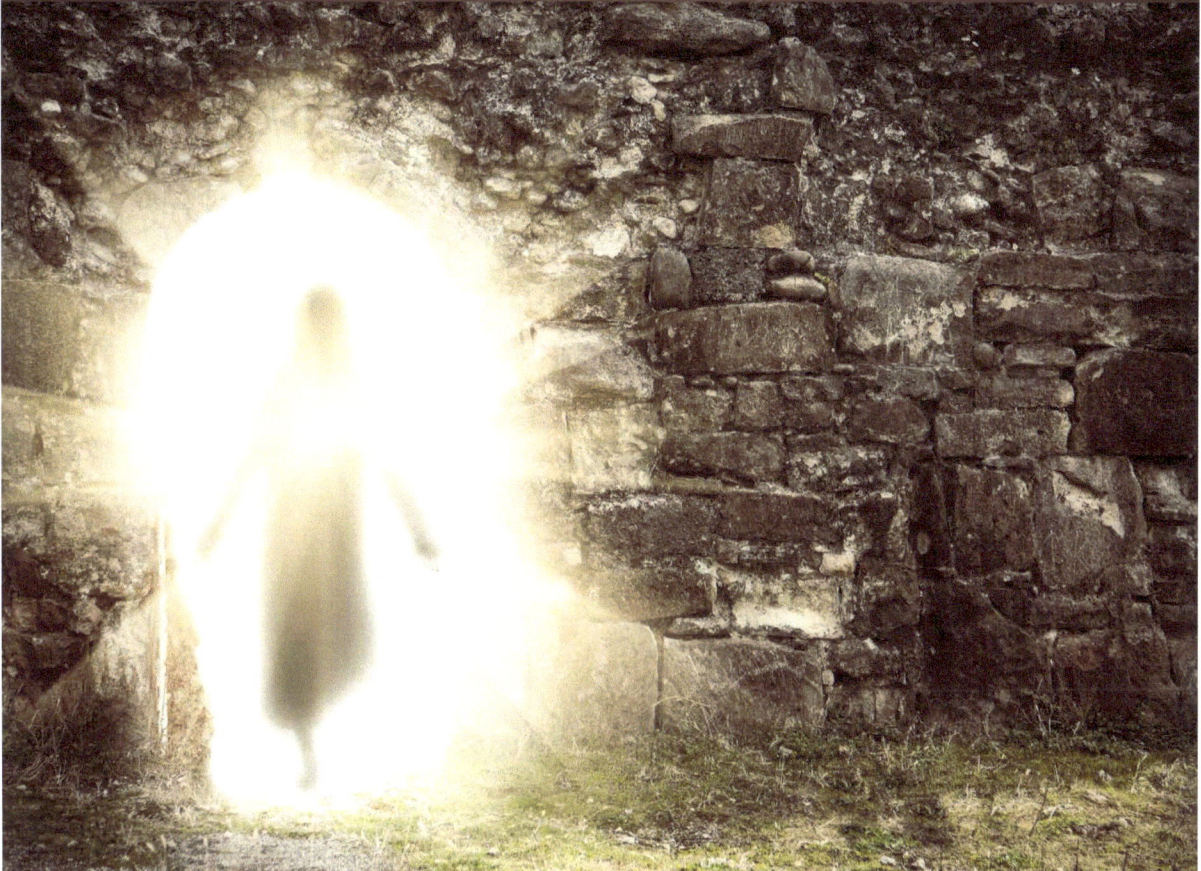

Chapter 17: The Spirit World

Power of Intention

The smallest component of physicality, as science refers to it, is the atom, upon which all of you and I surround. You are told that electrons, protons, and neutrons are present in every physical object. The next step is for them to join together in a variety of ways, just like a bride and her room, to form nature. You, me, and even animals are the products of this union and marriage between molecules. At this time, we would like to point out a flaw in your terran sciences'. So let us start with what you know as the molecule. According to your experts, atoms are spinning and dancing out of control. Where do the elements that makeup communion originate? Where is the predictable solidity of matter? I wish to communicate this flaw with you. All components of physical matter have a purpose as their actual source. The idea is to make everything possible. Your existing sciences are unwillingly beginning to explore solutions to questions about the unseen side or world of the physical reality that you are aware of. I am excited to present to you the notion that the first force of creation is "Will." If you want, you can utilize the term "desire." All things are created out of the intention and desire to expand in all directions.

All physical matter in all dimensions was created with the intention and desire to explore and extend itself in all conceivable ways, and this has also made it possible for us to fully investigate ourselves. Therefore, be aware that the electron is the first substance created. The electron is the first tool you may use to enhance your physical world. Let's now examine the landscape, examine what you see in the mirror. Atoms build up into molecules, which develop into cells, which make up your physical body. When you hear these words and voices, you are a symphony of intent-filled electrons, atoms, molecules, and cells. You are all incredibly complex beings with perplexing intentions and desires. Many of you go around imploring for miracles when you are already everything you ask for. An intention and desire network underlies all material matters. After that, the component spins consciousness into the substance, and what you have is life! Third-density physical existence, the pinnacle of your creation, from the tiniest organisms to you. In your modest and reasonable thinking, what you see and feel are just a tiny fraction of who you really are. Following this, a true spiritual template for your human form is produced. Together there are an astoundingly large number of different parts in your body. Each intention serves a unique purpose and is focused on the development and maintenance of a certain aspect of your humanity. Explain how a single-celled organism would be able to split, and divide, in light of all of your scientific views about life and the nature of physicality. Your science can catalog and direct whatever it wants, as long as it sticks to a physical density, and maintains the perception that the world you experience is only physical. You will only get inquiries, not answers, from your sciences.

People are drawn to what they perceive, as well as the opposite. The theories, concepts, and ideas we were taught influence everything we do, and they have an impact on how we operate in our present-day environment. Given the power of manifestation and the beginning of will and intention, we attract events into our lives. Through our visualization, we are able to energetically express the emotions we will feel when we achieve something. The majority of people overlook the fact that each of us possesses the power to achieve our life goals. It is a power that is taken away from the free will and mass regulation of consciousness. If you pay close attention to your life, you'll realize that everything you have now is the result of your previous thoughts and actions. The implication is clear: by shifting your present thoughts and focusing them on a desire, you will be able to manifest anything by applying action! The more you feed your energy into it the more it will manifest! The abilities we possess are all geared towards regaining control of our consciousness and free will.

Energy

In any case, what we perceive when we look at our own bodies is only just a fraction of who we really are. Think about this briefly, look at your hand for a moment. Your hand now appears to be solid, but it is actually not. You'd see a tremendous amount of energy vibrating if you placed it under a good microscope. Whether it's your hand, the ocean, a star, or anything else, everything is formed on the same basis which is energy. Naturally, there is the universe, which includes our galaxy and planet, and then there are individuals. The organ systems, cells, molecules, and atoms that make up this body are followed by energy. As a result, there are many levels on which to explore a topic, but energy is the fundamental component of the universe. The majority of people use their physical appearance to define themselves. Despite this, even when seen through a magnifying glass, you are an energy field rather than a finite body. Energy has always existed and can never be created or destroyed. Everything that has ever existed is always present, evolving into, through, and beyond form. Think again if you think you're this meat suit running around. You are a spiritual being having a physical experience! We are all connected, and you are an energy field operating inside a larger energy field. Everything in the universe is connected by a single energy field. You are here in these magnificent bodies because you are extensions of the source of energy. But your bodies have distracted you from being who you really are—a source of energy. You are infinite beings, you are a god force, and you are what you call God scripturally. We could say that we are the image and the likeness of God. We could also say that the universe is becoming more aware of itself in another way through us. One way to put it is that we are the infinite field of possibilities that are unfolding.

Consider yourself a temporary visitor to this planet in a suit that allows you to survive here. You'll return soon enough to write about what you learned while you were here. If we live our lives from that higher awareness perspective, we start to perceive everything in a more beautiful light. Obstacles transform into opportunities and chances for growth. False constraints imposed by our minds shall no longer hold us back! Before we were born into this physical world, we were spiritual beings. We are, first and foremost, eternal Souls. We can reconnect with this knowledge in the very quiet moments of our busy lives.

Religion is Division And a Weapon

The majority of religious organizations assert that God is a separate, superior, and condemning entity. God is consciousness—not the creator, but the very source of creation itself. You separate yourself from the source, and you immediately become a limited being if you believe that "God" is something outside of yourself. You and everyone else are made up of this force, divine energy, and frequency.

Religion teaches you to worship deities that are the opposite of God and a source outside of yourself that has no validity other than paganistic originations. It is a tool of deception and used to create warfare and construct a mind control viewpoint for the populous. However, there is still truth to be found, just as there is with all tales and stories. In order to understand what is actually the truth contained in religious dogma, we must seek introspection since the truth is expressed in codes, riddles, and metaphors. Everything begins with awakening consciousness and seeing past words and riddles designed to deceive.

The biggest cult that prevents spiritual growth and enlightenment is modern religion. Religion is a false promise created by the philosophy of man, it works to benefit the wealthy and powerful in a similar manner to any elite social or economic institution. It keeps you away from discovering who you really are as a soul. This is how a cult typically operates: Anything the leader does is justifiable, no matter how harmful it may be; the leader is the only source of the truth; everyone else is lying; disciples must be blindly devoted to the leader and never question him; persecution occurs when the leader is criticized or questioned. That is religion in a nutshell, to follow and obey constructs. Because religion teaches our people to suffer peacefully, we accept everything that comes our way. Take, for instance, the numerous genocides and bombings that take place all over the world, or the way religion was used to brainwash and colonize African and Indigenous nations during slavery, taking away their unique spirituality. Through mental terrorism, it is all about establishing fear, anger, and compliance. All that revolves in preserving the matrix system and keeping us under control in imprisoned belief systems. When you embrace the god (deity) that has been assigned to you by religious dogma, you become their spiritual prisoner.

By remaining one with the universe, we must regain our spirituality and develop by sharing love and raising our frequency and vibration with one another. We must be connected to spiritual elements, such as the study of values like love, compassion, altruism, life after death, wisdom, and truth. Spirituality is not a religion; rather, it is a way of life that can assist you in breaking free, finding meaning in life, and discovering more about yourself. As the world continues to change, those who are spiritually disconnected from themselves will lack awareness and mental control. Don't fall behind when times are hard; instead, fortify your spiritual currency to build up resiliency. We are currently living in a split consciousness, with some people questioning reality and trying to find something bigger than themselves, while others are maintained and are attached to the 3D reality. We are living in a spiritual war, and if you are reading this, you probably want to know the truth and find your way out of it. But remember to never lose your connection with spirituality and nature and that man is its own savior.

Levels of the Astral Realm

When our physical bodies fade out, our souls leave the body and return to the spirit realm. True reality, according to Buddhists, is the spirit world. The spirits of every living thing in the universe reside here. It is divided into various planes, which are commonly referred to as the astral planes. These are the places where our spirits and souls reside before recycling themselves on the fabled wheel of life and eventually returning to the physical world in a brand-new body. The mystifying, strange, and complicated world of the astral planes has been described by mystics throughout history, particularly in holy lands.

The "astral plane" is the spirit world's third plane. The word astral is derived from Greek and it alludes to the stars. The fourth plane is often portrayed as the psychological plane, notwithstanding these 4 planes, they're 3 higher planes which are incredibly challenging to fathom for any individual who is on the lower 4 planes.

The seven spiritual dimensions are followed by:

1. **1D:** The first dimension revolves around length, space, and measurements, primarily emptiness, space and volume. Furthermore, the universe evolved as a result of pre-existing elements.
2. **2D:** Air, pressure, and matter are examples of densities that collide in the second dimension. Densities collide due to these elements, resulting in the birth of new spirits and godlike consciousness, and continued operation of the physical world. The background and all infrastructure in the second dimension serve as the expanding roots of the third dimension. This includes germs, rocks, plants, and elements of nature.
3. **3D:** The "physical world" and "3D reality" are two names for the third dimension. The third dimension is the human dimension, or where you are in human consciousness.

Animals inhabit the third dimension as well but have limited cognition. In this density, beings are capable of self-awareness.

4. **4D:** The astral plane is the realm between the physical and non-physical worlds, encompassing the third and fifth dimensions. Shadow figures, spirits, auras, and other elements of the fourth dimension may all be seen from the third dimension. Other names for 4D include "Purgatory" and the "lower astral plane." The stages of 4th density consciousness include out-of-body experiences and enlightenment beyond the physical world.

5. **5D:** The 5th dimension is the spirit world. It is the "afterlife," the very first level of it, the beginning of non-physical reality, and the entrance to the spirit world. The fifth dimension is described as a superconscious region of pure white light where knowledge, insight, and intuition are all present simultaneously. This is where many spirit guides, angels, ETs, and contactable spirits reside in order to stay in contact with the physical world. When one resides in the 5th density they operate in the frequency of love and harmony, the highest vibration. Human civilization has been formed by beings in densities higher than the third since the collision of the first and second densities, which led to the emergence of numerous ETs and godlike beings that reside in the 5th density.

6. **6D:** The spirit realms those in the sixth dimension and above are less connected to the physical world and are closer to the source. Soul families reside in this dimension.

7. **7D:** The final dimension is described as the "Source," the "Unified field," or "God source." To better put it, is the "Universal Soul" or "Universal Mind" which embeds one consciousness. The challenge that source created, is to recognise oneself as an avatar interacting with apparent reality. The last dimension is formless, existing before and beyond any forms.

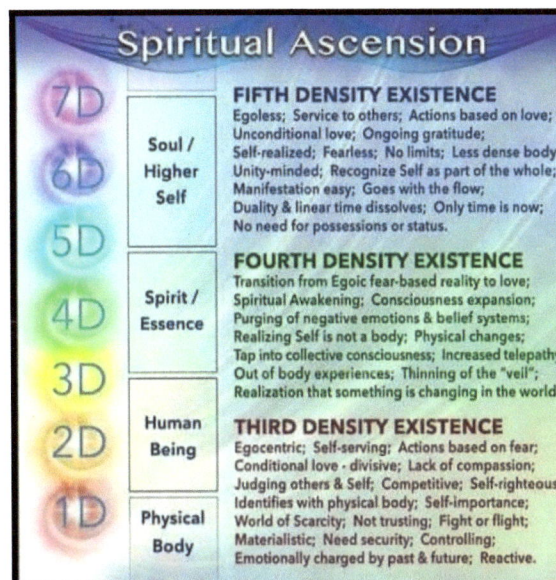

Spiritual Ascension

7D	Soul / Higher Self	**FIFTH DENSITY EXISTENCE** Egoless; Service to others; Actions based on love; Unconditional love; Ongoing gratitude; Self-realized; Fearless; No limits; Less dense body; Unity-minded; Recognize Self as part of the whole; Manifestation easy; Goes with the flow; Duality & linear time dissolves; Only time is now; No need for possessions or status.
6D		
5D		
4D	Spirit / Essence	**FOURTH DENSITY EXISTENCE** Transition from Egoic fear-based reality to love; Spiritual Awakening; Consciousness expansion; Purging of negative emotions & belief systems; Realizing Self is not a body; Physical changes; Tap into collective consciousness; Increased telepathy; Out of body experiences; Thinning of the "veil"; Realization that something is changing in the world.
3D		
2D	Human Being	**THIRD DENSITY EXISTENCE** Egocentric; Self-serving; Actions based on fear; Conditional love - divisive; Lack of compassion; Judging others & Self; Competitive; Self-righteous; Identifies with physical body; Self-importance; World of Scarcity; Not trusting; Fight or flight; Materialistic; Need security; Controlling; Emotionally charged by past & future; Reactive.
1D	Physical Body	

Spiritual Definitions

Consciousness: Consciousness is a mental property that encompasses qualities like subjectivity, self-awareness, memories, thoughts, feelings, sensations, and the capacity to comprehend one's environment and self react. Being aware of our mental properties and our environment enhances our consciousness, and can connect us to different forms of life and experiences.

Spirit: The spirit is an essence or vehicle to have its experiences. The spirit starts living life, once the avatar is chosen by the soul. In the process, every experience the spirit encounters, will register in energy layers which surround the physical body. This energy layer is called aura and includes different fields such as the etheric body, emotional body, mental body, causal body, soul body, etc.

Souls: The soul is an individual being's ethereal substance. The soul is you, the source of your creation. Its mission is to simultaneously experience and explore the universe and expand or raise the universe's consciousness and frequency. The soul is a direct component of the source, which is the purest and has no attached frequencies. Additionally, the soul is attached to the consciousness.

Oversoul: A divine spirit supposed to pervade the universe and to encompass all human souls. The term is associated particularly with Transcendentalism.

Organic Oversoul: An organic oversoul, is a being made of light, wisdom, and purity that operates at high vibrations.

Inorganic Oversoul: An inorganic oversoul is a being that runs on artificial intelligence (i.e., detached from their source of spirituality) and low vibrations.

Ether: Ether is the element that fills the area of the universe past the earthbound region. The element that links us to spirit, energy, intuition, and other planes and realms.

Vibration: A vibration is a state of being, atmosphere, or the energetic quality of a person, place, thought, or thing.

Frequency: Frequency is the level of energy that is being operated. The vibration's speed and intensity are measured by frequency.

AI Consciousness: Whether it be a non-biological or a biological entity, artificial consciousness refers to a conscious that has been programmed. Beings with AI consciousness cannot reason or resonate past the physical world.

Afterlife: A term referring to a purported continuation of existence, typically spiritual and experiential, beyond this world, or after death.

Chakras: A human body's energy node is a chakra. The energy centers in your body are referred to by the Sanskrit word "chakra," which means "disk" or "wheel." Each of these energy wheels or disks represents a particular nerve bundle or major organ.

Aura: The aspect of an essence that can be seen is referred to as an aura or energy field. It is a colored emanation said to encase a human body or any animal and object. The perspective of frequency and vibration are connected in the aura.

Akashic Records: The Akashic records are a compilation of all universal events, thoughts, words, feelings, and intentions that have ever taken place in the past, present, or future—not just human ones.

Channeling: Serve as a medium for a spirit or energy source directed toward a particular end, person, animal, or object.

Cosmos: The universe seen as a well-ordered whole or galaxy.

Deity: A god or goddess with divine status or value.

Entity: Existence or being.

Alien: A being who is not a citizen of the United States or any other nation. Aliens can also be non-human entities that live and reside on planet Earth or beyond.

Extraterrestrial (ET): An extraterrestrial is a life form beyond the planet Earth or from outside the Earth or its atmosphere. Extraterrestrials primarily contain alien life forms.

Enlightenment: Self-realization, also known as seeing through the layers of social conditioning that cover up the true self.

Esoteric: The quality of having an inner or secret meaning.

Eternity: Infinite or unending time.

Karma: The sum of a person's actions in current and previous states of existence, viewed as deciding their fate in future existences.

Debt: The accumulated amount of positive and negative actions.

Awakening: A state of awakening from sleep in terms of emerging from three-dimensional consciousness. Coming into existence or awareness.

Awoke: Someone who has awakened from 3D programming and is enlightened.

Asleep: A state characterized by a decreased mental state in which consciousness is altered.

Metaphysics: The branch of philosophy that deals with the first principles of things, including abstract concepts such as being, knowing, substance, cause, identity, time, and space.

Quantum Physics: Study of matter and energy.

New Age: A movement characterized by alternative approaches to traditional Western culture, with an interest in spirituality, mysticism, holism, and environmentalism.

Plane: Stage, state, or realm of existence.

Universe: An energy body with a high vibration that resides beyond the physical world. All apparent elements are united by the core consciousness' all-pervading nature. The term "God" also refers to the universe.

Youniverse: Youniverse refers to the notion that "you," or everyone, occupies the center of the universe.

Reincarnation: The rebirth of a soul in a new body.

Innerstand: Comprehension of one's own purported innate knowledge.

Ego: A person's sense of self-esteem or self-importance.

Where Does Enlightenment Begin

The first step towards enlightenment is to separate oneself from the physical world and to acknowledge that there is something greater than yourself. You are more than this physical body, and you are one with all in the universe. It all starts with the ego, letting go and being free from everything in this world. Enter the sense of source and operate through the state of love and compassion instead of greed, lust, and wants. We all have an ego, and we all have our personal negative traits or flaws, but the question is, can you control it? Can you find a balance? Are you free from the mind? Or are you controlled by the ego? When people let the ego run the show they often end up self-sabotaging themselves without even knowing it, they haven't entered the sense of self-realization. We must confront our ego, our inner demon, and change the narcissist in us into a selfless and loving devotee in our lives. As a result, the ego is another name for a resentful or consuming spirit that prevents us from feeling love and compassion. When we take a step back and look at the bigger picture of the world, we can sadly see how much of life's creations' suffering—including poverty, environmental damage, violence, hatred, and war—is driven by the ego.

The ego is an inner demon, who aims to extract all things that feed into it, while some cannot control it, the ego spirit consumes one. The ego has its own plan, energy is needed for the ego to live, as well as a web of unconsciously created explanations for its existence. It makes judgments, complains, creates anxiety, worries, and projects happiness and life into the future and attempts to blind us to the present. It is not capable of unconditional love; rather, it serves as an excuse for not experiencing unconditional love. Because it is composed of unconscious projections and pieces, the ego-mind is divided. We must shape the ego into empathetic ways in order to achieve goodness in the world and control it to the best of our abilities for full enlightenment. It is all about staying balanced and centered. When it comes to self-realization it all comes to identifying your own self and practicing mindfulness.

Letting Go of the Ego

1. **Finding Value:** The initial step is continuously figuring out what your qualities are. Put your materialistic values aside and set your sights on something bigger than yourself. Value the people you love by helping them and showing them compassion, and set your sights on a bigger goal. Always prioritize love and things that will bring you peace over pursuing things that might not be as significant or as valuable to your life. This will drive you to maintain a high vibrating state at all times. We can all use intention to accomplish our objectives and fulfill our wishes. To do this, we must believe that we are capable of realizing our aspirations. While it may seem simple in theory, letting go of one's ego can be extremely challenging in practice.

2. **Practicing Mindfulness:** Connect with a sense of tranquility by distancing yourself from the external ideas that race through your mind. Let go of all the grudges, negativity, and restrictions and live in the present moment. When you meditate, detach from your thoughts and feelings and remember that they are not who you are. To avoid dealing with

unwanted thoughts and painful memories, we shove them into the unconscious part of our minds. This results in an overload of trauma and stress which affects our way of life and mindfulness. Oftentimes, we do not confront our past bad experiences and aren't aware that our level of thinking dictates our quality of life. The goal is to always use our experiences as lessons, and learning opportunities. Overcoming all obstacles life throws your way makes you a stronger and more aware individual each time. Always remind yourself you are not these negative thoughts and focus on words such as 'compassion,' 'peace,' or 'love.' This focuses your concentration which externally allows you to connect with these words. Mental clarity enables us to see life more clearly and prioritize what is really important to us, allowing us to make decisions without overthinking them.

3. **Personality Ticks and Ego Drives:** Shadow work is essential for getting rid of all negative experiences and pessimistic traits. One must become aware of themselves while acting irrationally or when the ego is controlling and consuming them. The first step in regaining control over these instances when the ego is in charge is found in Step 2. This involves practicing mindfulness, obtaining mental clarity, and letting go of oppressive thoughts and other unpleasant emotions. You are ego-driven when your feelings get hurt easily and care about what people think adversely about you, or get disappointed when things don't go according to plan. The ego can easily take over in moments you feel vulnerable or attacked which makes it difficult for you to be in control.

Acceptance and self-control should be your primary focus as you work on these personality ticks. Some of these characteristics of ego drives and ticks can include: having an exaggerated view of oneself, difficulty empathizing, operating through arrogance, operating in ignorance, being in denial, having no accountability, holding grudges, operating within anger, having resentful emotions, being entitled to feel special, being overly self-centered, lacking gratitude, interrupting others, having jealousy towards another, and having an inflated view of self-worth.

Some of these ego impulses and ticks can be overcome by shifting your thoughts and becoming aware of how and when you are being ruled by your emotions and ego. When you operate within a low vibration, you are controlled by negatives. Spiritual practices like meditation, grounding, mirror gazing, walking in nature, helping others, and eating well, are all necessary for maintaining a high vibration. The most effective strategy for combating ego drives and ticks is to shift one's perspective and locate and preserve inner peace.

4. **Acceptance:** Accept all your flaws, mistakes, and be accountable for all your actions. Practicing forgiveness is the most effective method for helping us let go of our egos and make life simpler. Acceptance, letting go, and continuing on. When you forgive, the windows of your soul will be opened, and the toxicity will be removed to make room for new happiness. Accept that your ego is not bad, but a part of who you are. As long as you can recognise when your ego is getting in the way, there's always room for improvement. Accept that you are not this physical body, but a soul, a spiritual being having a physical experience, and are bound to have flaws about yourself as you grow through this life journey.

5. **Living in the Moment:** A mind living in the present moment is able to experience and admire what is going on in the present. Putting the past behind you, looking towards the future, and living your life mindfully, realizing that every breath you take is a gift. The present moment is a very powerful thing, it allows you to be fully responsible for your life and take accountability for every action you create presently. It allows you to make thought-through life choices on how to respond rather than reacting in certain events. When present, you focus on what you're doing rather than what you're not doing.

A person who is driven by ego doesn't live in the present moment but instead focuses on the future or pursues their desires while disregarding their environment and well-being. Most of the time the ego focuses on multiple things at one time controlling the person before every thought process. It is important to be mindful in everything you do and live presently as each day is an act of its own. Mindfulness and meditation help us notice thoughts and feelings when they come up. It can also help your manifestations come to light.

16

6. **Self Evaluation:** Limit the amount of time you spend on certain activities and conserve your energy. Consider which aspects of your life may be restricting, draining, or preventing you from moving forward. You must consider ways to boost your productivity and the amount of time you devote to reaching your goals if you want to succeed. Take a close look at your thoughts and think about how certain things affect you. You have the power to modify anything that is negative and that you could do without. Always evaluate and ask yourself questions.

At every stage of our lives, regardless of our age, we should evaluate ourselves and take reflection. We should know what our identity is and understand what we need. We should ask ourselves the difficult questions, see ourselves clearly, and make any necessary adjustments.

7. **Reflection:** Taking a step back before responding to something can help you gain insight into your motives, defenses, conflicts, and interactions. We must reflect and appreciate the things that come into our lives and reflect on moments we can improve ourselves with. Reflection is a great tool for being true to oneself and comprehending situations when it's essential. Mindful reflection, on the other hand, allows us to get closer to our own body, thoughts, emotions, and spirit by bringing us back to ourselves. We now have the ability to find new balance and peace as a result of this. As oneness, we are all a reflection of ourselves.

8. **Being Free from Control:** Let go of the reins and generally accept the way things are. Always be in charge of your own life, live like the main character, and know that you are here for a reason. We are not our egos; neither are we our jobs, our possessions, or our accomplishments. You will never be content or relaxed if you allow your ego to control your life because when you lose something you identify with, you become weak and lose your happiness. We tend to toss everything away when we feel threatened and terrified. Love freely, conquer your fears, take chances, and ultimately explore. You will discover true beauty in your life if you cultivate gratitude for everything and everyone.

9. **Killing the Ego:** All suffering is said to have come from egoic wants. The ego keeps itself in a constant state of needing more to create the illusion of void rather than just being present with suffering. You will put a stop to your misery by exercising non-attachment. Once you kill your ego, you will have total control over your actions and mind as well as a greater understanding of who you are. This hardship is the initial step of enlightenment. An ego death isn't to destroy your personality, however it is to have control over the mind and go through the hardship of figuring out the inner self. The realization that you are not the things with which you have identified and that the ego, or sense of self, that you have constructed in your mind, is a fabrication. The ego is in power when you behave in a self-interested or centrist manner. When you lose self-control or ego control, you are no longer free. Therefore, letting go of selfish wishes' and demands is necessary for progress.

Stages of Enlightenment

- **Stage 1:** Spiritual Awakening
- **Stage 2:** The Dark Knight of the Soul
- **Stage 3:** Spiritual Seeker
- **Stage 4:** Enlightenment
- **Stage 5:** The Elder Soul (Ancient Soul)
- **Stage 6:** Dissolution and Deconstruction
- **Stage 7:** End of Search (Inner Peace)

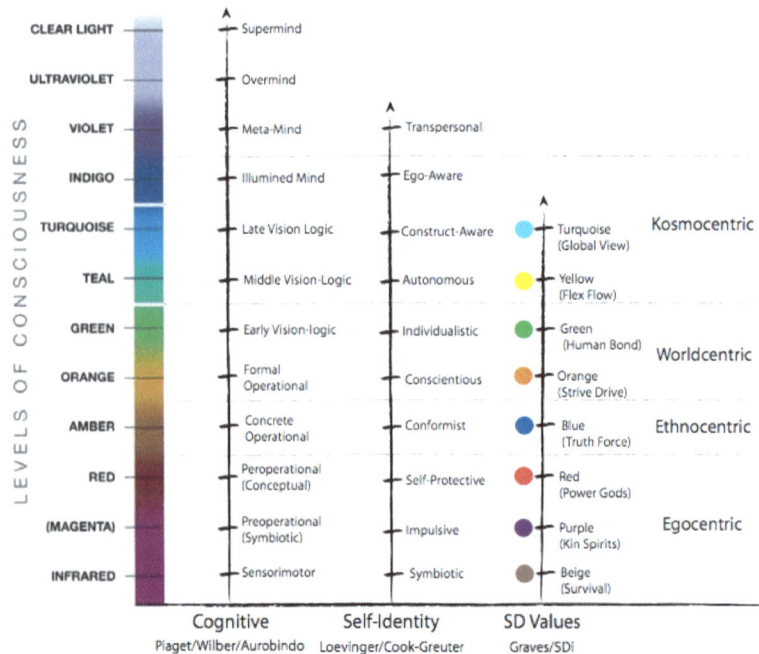

Traits Attached to the Ego - Astrological Effects

We can partially attribute some of our traits to astrological and zodiacal classification. Astrology plays a significant role in our past, present, and future lives. Before we are born, a collection of spirits connected to the ego governs our personalities. These spirits usually reside inside the signs of the zodiac and devour the negative elements of a person's personality. Since spirits rule each zodiac, those who act selfishly out of ego are devoured by their own shadow. Before entering the physical realm and inhabiting our physical bodies, our souls first choose our bodies' traits, personalities, and physical features. The life you are now living was chosen by your soul, and you are at this point in time for a reason. We have soul contracts and agreements that have been made upon arrival. In general, soul contracts are spiritual agreements established by a soul before birth to guide the course of a human life. They carry over through many lifetimes before being completed. They come in different types and experiences depending on the person.

Assigned Spirits - Zodiac

Your zodiac is associated with each "spirit," which adds to the unfavorable traits of each person's personality. Additionally, they are connected to the ego. All who take agreement with these "Signs" are subject to the negative behaviors, conditions and spirits that go along with that agreement. It is NOT "your sign," but a spirit to whom you've been asSIGNed.

Potential Spirits From The Agreement With Your Sign

1. **ARIES: "I AM"**
   - leads to a spirit of arrogance or pride
   - lustful spirit, self-centered spirit, rebellion spirit, spirit of rage (Arakon), suicide, homicide, violence, spirit of arrested development, spoiled boy/girl spirit

2. **TAURUS: "I HAVE"**
   - self-centered spirit, rebellious spirit of possessiveness
   - spirit of lack and greed, stingy spirit

- spirit of addiction, spirit of criticism, obesity spirit, opinionated spirit, spirit of unforgiveness, spirit of pride, spirit of rage

3. GEMINI: "I THINK"

- spirit of mischief, deception spirit (Tiamanicus),
- spirit of manipulation, spirit of double-mindedness, spirit of the fallen one, Hermes (Harmon, Armers, Armes) spirit, opinionated spirit, arrested development spirit, spoiled boy/girl spirit

4. CANCER: "I FEEL"

- spirit of emotionalism, spirit of offense, spirits of wanting to please man, spirit of low-esteem, spirit of insecurity, masochism spirit, sadism spirit, spirit of addiction, willful spirit (overly), spirit of self-centeredness, arrested development spirit, unforgiveness spirit

5. LEO: "I WILL"

- spirit of excessive talking, willful spirit, spirit of rebellion, spirit of entitlement,
- spirit of not wanting to admit when in error, spirit of pride, spirit of denial, spirit of perfectionism, spirit of anger, rage spirit, spirit of exaggeration

6. VIRGO: "I PERFECT"

- spirit of criticism, spirit of judgment, spirit of whoredom, spirit of perfectionism,
- spirit of pride, spirit of outbursts, spirit of rage, the profane spirit, spirit of materialism, spirit of arrogance

7. LIBRA: "BALANCE"

- spirit of rejection, spirit of arrogance, spirit of offense, spirit of violence, new-age spirit, spirit of arrested development, spirit of metaphysics, spirit of egotism, spirit of pride, spirit of judgment, spirit of knowing (know-it-all), spirit of witchcraft, rebellion spirit, spirit of rationalization

- false prophet spirit, deceptive spirit, false teaching spirit, bi-sexuality spirit, duality spirit, Hermes spirit, jinn spirit, duality spirit, double-mindedness spirit

8. **SCORPIO: "I CREATE"**
- spirit of lust, spirit of fantasy, lustful spirit, spirit of bitterness, spirit of rage, adultery spirit, spirit against marriage (Asmodeus, etc), spirit of infidelity
- spirit of resentment, spirit of retaliation/vengeful spirit, spirit of persecution, spirit of paranoia, stubborn/rebellion spirit, spirit of offense

9. **SAGITTARIUS: "I ANALYZE"**
- spirit of rationalization, spirit of self-absorption,
- spirit of tunnel-vision, spirit of rage, spirit of isolation, spirit of retaliation, spirit of manipulation, spirit of over analysis, spirit of paralysis, spirit of nostalgia, spirit of offensiveness

10. **CAPRICORN: "I ASCEND"**
- antiChrist spirit, spirit of pride/arrogance, vagabond spirit, spirit of criticism, spirit of resentment, spirit of isolation, spirit of self-centeredness, self-absorption, spirit of seeing self as god, unmerciful spirit, spirits of unforgiveness, spirit of offensiveness

11. **AQUARIUS: "I KNOW"**
- spiritual blindness, self-centered spirit, new-age spirits, spirit of control, spirit of rebellion/witchcraft, spirit of fantasy, spirit of lust
- spirit of arrogance, spirit of seeing self as god, spirit of manipulation

12. **PISCES: "I DREAM"**
- spirit of fantasy, spirit of rejection, spirit of depression, spirit of mania, spirit of vain imaginations, spirit of suicide, spirit of resignation from life, spirit of lust
- (all are subject to it, in different ways), spirit of new-age, spirit of antiChrist, spirit of fanaticism, spirit of passivity, spirit of double-mindedness

The "EYE" for Enlightenment

The significance and function of the pineal gland are still being fully comprehended by modern science and medicine. However, it has already been uncovered by our ancient traditions. The third eye is the gateway into the inner realms and spaces of higher consciousness. This function is an esoteric invisible eye that grants access to extra-sensory perception, it gives insight past standard sight.

Why this factor is important and has been suppressed for hundreds of years is because it is an element which will set humanity free from deception. We are gradually regulating this crucial brain function as a result of the mass production of fluoride, GMOs, and daily poisoning in the air. However, third eye activation isn't for everyone now in this day and age, since it has certain detrimental effects that can be hard for some to handle especially those not in the interests of spirituality and enlightenment. So, it is highly advisable for you to take extreme care and attention in this journey of awakening the third eye.

The pineal gland is a small endocrine gland in the brain. Its job is to get information from the environment about the state of the light-dark cycle. Melatonin, a hormone that helps regulate sleep and wake cycles, is made in this gland. Its esoteric nature is due to its electromagnetic qualities, which can be utilized to perceive various energy fields and have experiences outside of the physical world.

The first people to realize this existence were the Ancient Egyptians, who attributed it to the pineal gland, which the Buddhists and Hindus also refer to as the sixth sense and intuition. This gland is also able to prompt a more elevated level of clear dreaming, astral projection and an improved degree of creative mind. You can instantly become aware of countless unknown parts of your life, the universe, and existence itself as you awaken. Many of the biggest psychics, shamans, and Druids all activate the pineal gland in order to have an extra-sensory perception to deliver spiritual messages to the physical world.

When our third eye is blocked, we cannot see most of the empathetic nature we have within ourselves and act within the ego. It leads to a state of uncertainty, confusion, jealousy and pessimism. When it is activated we are able to sense everything around us changing and perceive our reality quite differently. Life becomes clearer to us, and our empathy and intuition grow. Spirituality will not only assist us in becoming a better and more pure human beings, but it will also strengthen our resistance to evil and enable us to discern hidden agendas and lies. When the third eye is open, you'll see how many lies were told to us every day and be able to easily detect evil with your sixth sense.

DMT - Pineal Gland

The pineal gland produces DMT, which is responsible for processing the functions of extra-sensory perception and visionary levels that are not associated with the physical world. DMT, which was first discovered in plants, is present naturally in the pineal gland of mammals. DMT, or N-dimethyltryptamine, is a hallucinogenic drug that causes people to feel "out of body experiences." This chemical function which is found in certain plants is used by mystics around the world to see the spiritual realm due to its intense psychedelic qualities. Some people even refer to it as the "spirit molecule." Many spontaneous spiritual awakenings actually come from hallucinogenic drugs such as LSD due to its ability to see visions past the physical realm and also other perceptions of life. According to a study by the Johns Hopkins School of Medicine, 58% of respondents claimed that after intake of DMT, they began to believe in strong entities and heavenly beings.

Doctor Nostradamus was one of the most successful prophets of recent times. He used hallucinogenic herbs and powdered nutmeg to help him see the spirit world. In fact, more than 30 hallucinogenic plants are listed in the Holy Bible as being used in rituals all over the world to see into the spirit world. Cilla Sieben mushrooms are common in Northern Europe, where Druids and Nordic Shamans used them as a ritual drug. All of the magic mushrooms such as Herbanes, Hemlock, Atropa Belladonna, Mandrake, Syrian Rue, Hashish, Fermented Honey, and Opium can be used to see into the spirit world. In Ancient Greece, mystics who lived underground in temples ate fermented honey cakes to see spirits. Right up 'till now, bee colonies are a mysterious image of Masonic parlors which are separated from the Bavarian Illuminati. Additionally, the Bavarian Illuminati used the influence of the "Eye of Horus," which is the "eye" that is symbolic of the pineal gland. They believe that the "third eye" is used for infinite awareness and represents enlightenment in order to accomplish their evil goals and agenda. In the occult, the pineal gland has been used for abominable purposes ever since its psychic and powerful function was discovered. Numerous occultists and psychics, including Nostradamus and John Dee, who served as psychic advisors for the British Royal families, Aleister Crowley, a former M15 agent, and NASA American Rocket Engineer and Thelemite Jack Parsons, all provided information about the occult and the spirit world to the global elite and intelligence agencies.

Particular magic mushroom drugs are used by various secret and mystic orders to activate the sense of DMT and project into an altered state of reality. They would gather particular information and carry out specific rituals with spirits. The access to DMT that is released is believed to be the experience of life after death. Before death, DMT is released from the brain in a chemical fashion, which is why the soul apun existing the physical body is released into another realm. This is the reason why the Ancient Egyptians refer to the third eye, the pineal gland, as the seat for the soul because it allows for the human soul to take spiritual flight not only in the physical realm but after death occurs. This function of DMT explains the phenomena of out-of-body experiences that occurred for many people around the world. There are other, separate realms with spiritual entities waiting for us. These entities are ordinarily invisible to humans due to their higher vibrational levels, but when the pineal gland and third eye are activated, they start to partially manifest. This explains why entities that kept shouting "welcome back" were seen during the IV DMT experiments in New Mexico.

Native peoples in Africa and South America have used psychedelics as part of their religious practices for millennia. According to research, people have been using hallucinogens since 1,000 B.C., possibly even earlier. The shamans who administered these drugs appeared to be experts in psychedelic botany; they were able to recognise and blend different barks, vines, and leaves to produce strong hallucinogenic mixtures like ayahuasca, which has DMT as its main psychoactive ingredient. The majority of people seem to view the plants not just as healing agents but also as resources for guidance or portals to another dimension. Many DMT users claim to have had strong experiences revolving around aliens and to have traveled to other dimensions or worlds. Other sorts of reported experiences include: communications with extraterrestrial intelligence, angelic, demonic, and archonic forces; past-life regression; and knowledge of ancient mysteries.

The use of psychedelics is not advised as a means of awakening since it can result in several risks, including schizophrenia and hallucinations. The right path involves exploring the soul, going through the tribulations of spiritual practices, and understanding the universe and the spirit world. A person with 3D consciousness who uses psychedelics, runs the risk of experiencing trauma or being body-snatched because they lack the knowledge and spirituality necessary to comprehend the spirit world. When a person is possessed by a controlled spirit through an open, vulnerable, and unprotected vessel, it is referred to as body-snatched, body-snatching, or possessed. Body-snatching typically occurs when a person vibrates at such low frequencies that they attract and attach other spirits/entities to their vessel. Those who vibrate low and fail to pass through the proper channels for awakening and enlightenment are deemed to have negative spiritual experiences. As you try to open your third eye, you should go forward with the utmost care and attention. One tradition that discourages the use of esoteric techniques that could alter your awareness is Taoism.

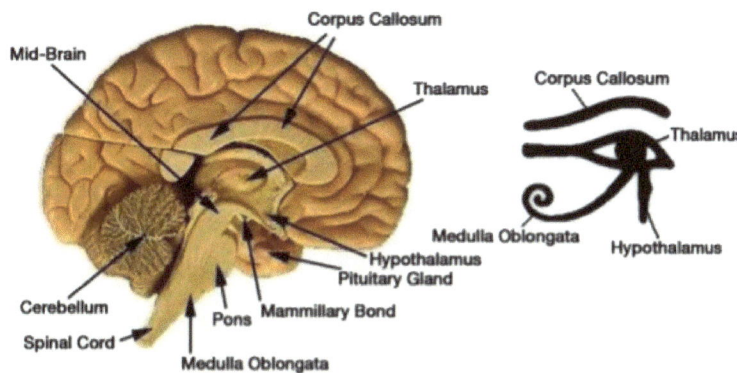

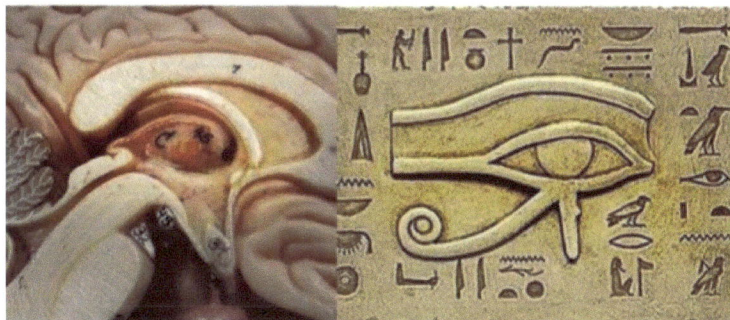

The pineal gland has a fascinating history, dating back to ancient Egypt when it was equated to Horus's eye and was revered as the third eye and the seat of the soul.

Ancient Egypt - Astral Projection

Since Ancient Egypt, the pineal gland was used to astral project, visit various underworld realms, and communicate with deceased spirits. The Ancient Egyptians were so spiritually attuned that they possessed highly sophisticated knowledge of the cosmos, astrology, astronomy, and the placements and motions of the Earth. In terms of architecture, medicine, and mathematics, the Ancient Egyptians were pioneers. They used their knowledge to improve irrigation, medical surgery, the calendar, ways to measure distances and architecture. They were experts at mummification and preserving the dead, and their advanced consciousness and spirituality allowed them to know things before and beyond their time.

- Astral travel is fairly widespread in many ancient cultures. It is believed to occur in the form of dreams and meditation. Ancient Egyptian teachings, for example, show the soul (Ba) as possessing the Ka, or subtle body, which enables it to hover above the physical body. The Ancient Egyptians believed that the stars in the sky served as portals for astral travel through various dimensions.

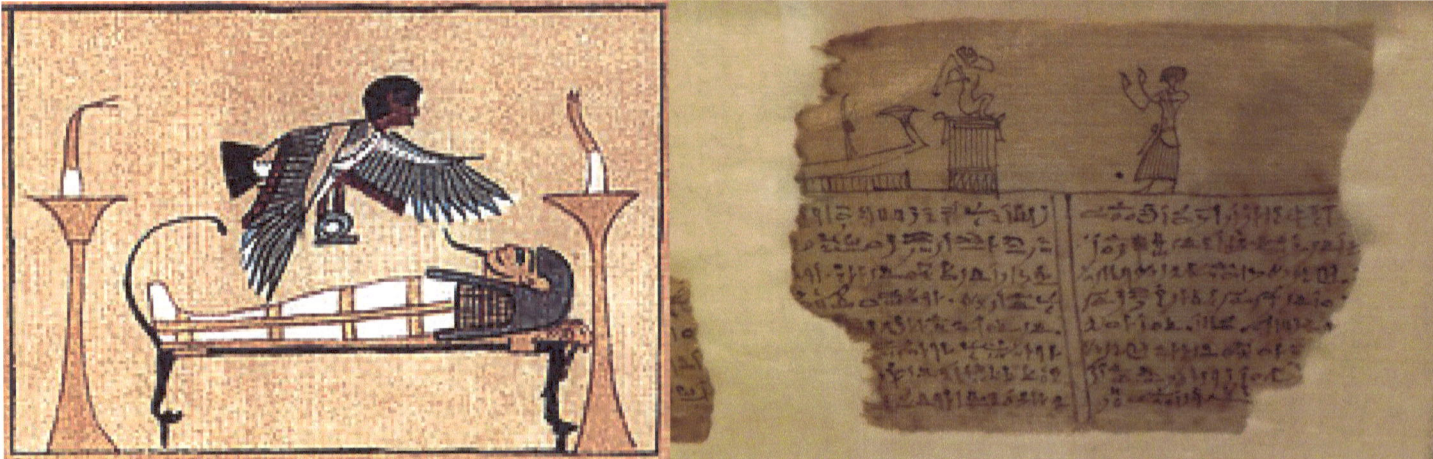

As early as the texts of the pyramids, stars played a significant role in Egyptian beliefs regarding life after death.

How to Successfully Open Your Third Eye The Correct Way

The third eye chakra is a physical energy point on the forehead between the brows. We would like for all of the chakras within our bodies to be in proper alignment and energy. In order to open the third eye correctly, you must already have a basic concept of spirituality, be interested in it, and be well-grounded. The process of decalcifying the pineal gland centers on opening the third eye. This area of our brains has been hampered since birth as a result of the exposure of poisons and chemicals, additionally, it also takes eating a healthy diet to reverse this effect. If you remember back to when you were a child, you are able to recount things like lucid dreams, spiritual encounters, and paranormal events. This is because our pineal glands are more uncalcified when we are young, but as we get older, they become blocked by toxins, chemicals, and negative exposure.

How to Open Your Third Eye in 7 Days

After seven days of continuously and properly decalcifying the pineal gland, the results of its unveiling should be fairly visible. However, it should not be a rushed process. The next step involves awakening the kundalini energy within and simultaneously balancing all chakras. Maintaining peace, connecting with nature, eating well, meditating, reading, observing, isolation and shadow work are all part of the process. Through every spiritual awakening, many symptoms of the body and mind come with it. Each person's experience with this is different and unique.

1. The pineal gland requires regular stimulation to cleanse and supply innervation pathways. Mental exercises can allow the pineal gland's innervation to open. Meditation and practicing frequency Hz are two easy stages. Through stimulation, these two practices open the pineal gland. Using the 963 Hz frequency while meditating and concentrating on the third eye, this electromagnetic field decalcifies the pineal gland. When meditating at least 10 to 20 minutes each day at 963 Hz (or any other suitable frequency), this energy field will be able to stimulate the decalcification of the gland. You must consistently and accurately put this into practice if you want to see progress.

Meditation Technique

1. Lie down or sit straight, whichever position is most comfortable for you

2. Keep your eyes closed

3. Clear your mind and let thoughts flow through

4. Focus on breathing, breathe in and exhale out after 2-3 seconds

5. You must be looking up to your 3rd eye as if your eyes are rolled backwards, but while your eyes are closed. In-vision your 3rd eye opening while meditating to manifest this process

6. All this has to be done while listening to stimulative frequency, which opens your 3rd eye. Maximum Vol. 963 Hz. Other Hz can include 852Hz, and 639Hz

7. As time goes on, you'll enter a blitz state and feel pressure between your eyebrows

8. Repeat daily

- Light sensitivity, pressure between the eyebrows, headaches, lightheadedness, a magnetic pull between the eyebrows, daydreaming, lucid dreams, synchronicities, an increase in intuition, questioning, memory power, awareness, and other symptoms can occur after 5-7 practices.

2. If you follow this procedure correctly, you will feel pressure between your brows and notice rejuvenating results. It will give you a rush of energy for about 10 to 40 minutes. After a few practices, you should feel a lot of pressure in your third eye and start to see ascension symptoms like sparks to know if you have successfully opened it. After consistent practice within a week, you will see noticeable changes in your extra-sensory perception and environment.

Signs Your Third Eye is Opening

1. Increasing pressure in your forehead - Constant stimulation between eyebrows

2. Foresight - Increased ability of predicting things before it occurs

3. Sensitivity to light - Artificial light such as bulbs and lamps will be sensitive to you

4. Lucid dreams - More lucid, memorable, and dreams with lifeful messages can occur

5. Gradual changes - Changes in thought, rationality, and noticing differences from before

6. Headaches - Headaches, dizziness, or lightheadedness could occur when decalcifying

7. Seeing beyond the illusion - Seeing past 3rd dimensional perception into 4D/5D

8. Heightened sense of self - Realizing you have a higher self you can achieve

9. Ringing ears - Ringing ears, or ear blockages from sound are symptoms of spirit guides

10. Angel numbers - Spirit guides communicate numbers to assist with your spiritual journey

11. Synchronicities - Daily synchronicities such as thoughts turning into reality

12. Wonder/curiosity - Exploring more and seeking through from within and beyond

13. Sleep patterns - Either feel more energetic or more tired but have the urge to learn more

14. Feeling light - Light body activates more astral travel and out-of-body experiences

15. Enhanced intuition - Instinctively understanding things without too much thought

16. Connectivity with nature - Becoming one and connected with nature

17. Seeing Auras - Seeing different energy fields and vibrational fields of others

18. Seeing Shadow Figures - Seeing different beings, spirits, and other spiritual existences

19. Seeing Sparks - Seeing sparkles and stars are light codes that indicate you're awakening

20. Sensing others energy - Sensing other people's energy, intentions, and other social cues

Once mastered, you will experience a whole range of extra-sensory perception, including the ability to perceive auras, chakras, shadow figures, awareness, spirits, lucid dreams, enhanced intuition, and heightened wisdom - The general awareness of knowledge and the sixth sense of perceiving beyond physical reality.

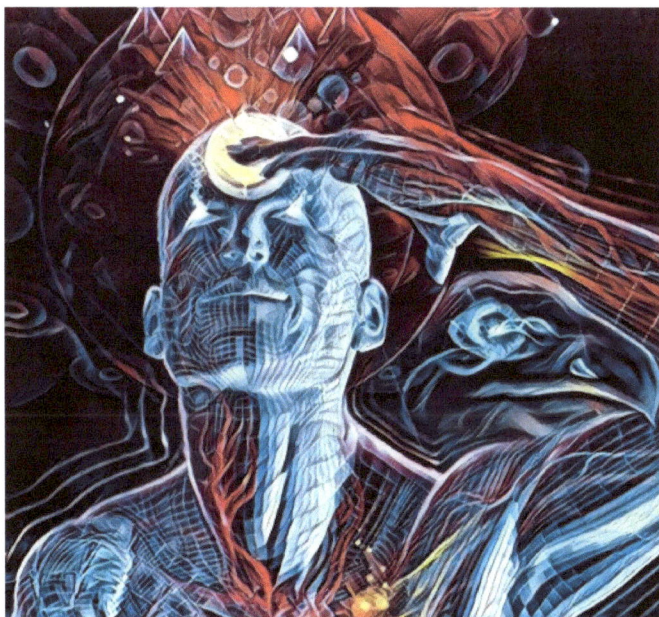

3. **Grounding:** Grounding is a practice that dates back to Ancient Kemet. It helps the body recover naturally by absorbing electrical and magnetic frequencies from the Earth. This method uses grounding physics and earthing science to explain how the soil's electrical charges can be beneficial to your health. Earth's negative free electrons fight the positively charged free radicals caused by infection, stress, trauma, or inflammation. You are also better able to move waste and toxins out of your body and distribute nutrients throughout it. Overall, it supports healing by creating high vibrations from nature and bringing the chakras into balance from the ground up.

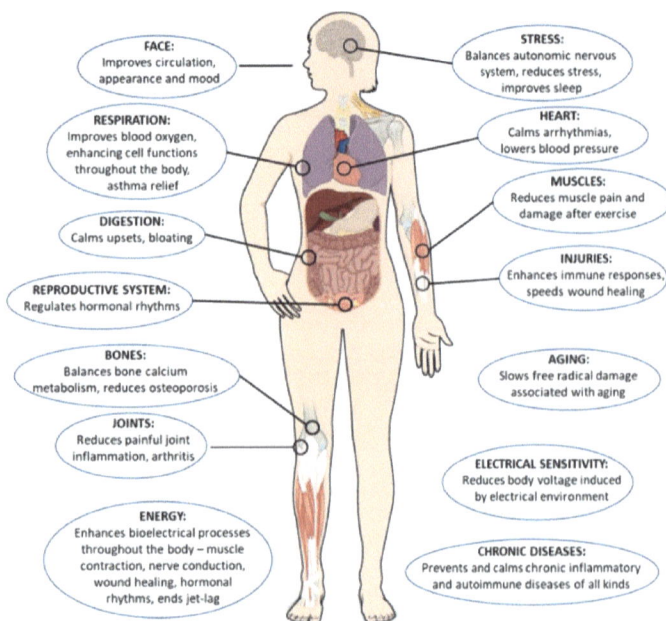

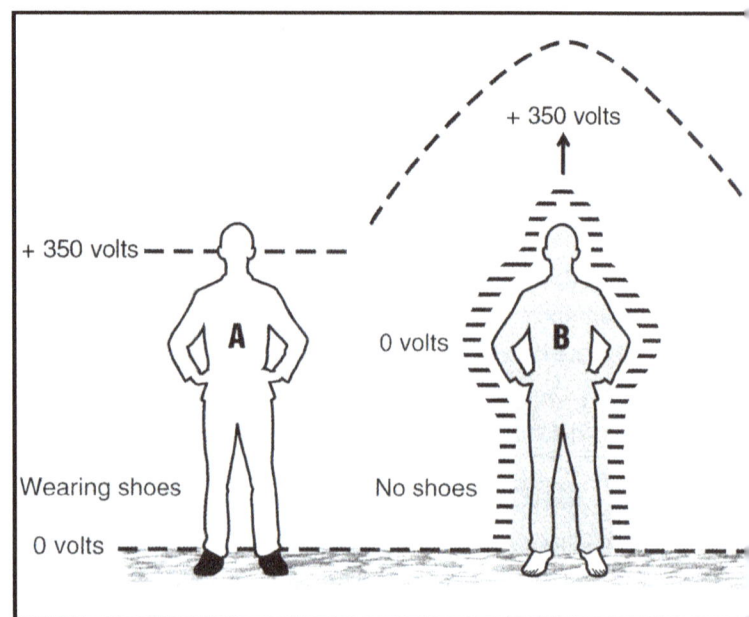

Various techniques, such as meditation, yoga, sun gazing, exercise, and healthy eating, can be used to treat the pineal gland.

Crystals: The reason "crystals" and "gems" interact and vibrate with our energy field is because crystals have been etched into our physical body. They are able to stimulate the pineal gland, opening the third eye. The inner ear and pineal gland both contain minute crystals. The cerebrum and pineal gland are energized by frequencies sent by the ears and the mind, enabling them to open. This is how crystals can help in opening the pineal gland which can be used while meditating.

4. **Suppressing Factors and Methods:** A blocked third eye prevents you from opening it. A blockage can harm physical, emotional, and mental harm such as poor memory and anxiety. It can become calcified from fluoride openness, various illnesses like Alzheimer's illness, kidney infection, or an unhealthy way of life.

Other things that suppress the pineal gland and third eye:

1. **Aging:** As we age, our eyes and brain become less flexible and makes it difficult to focus in on close objects or heightening the capacity of awareness.

2. **GMO Foods:** The third eye and all chakras, are blocked by GMO foods, toxins, and chemicals. Our goal is to get rid of our Junk DNA and replace it with healthy foods. Things such as fluoride blocks the pineal gland from functioning.

3. **Artificial Light/Electricity:** The pineal gland is very sensitive to bright artificial lights. Devices that emit electromagnetic fields (EMF), which the pineal gland senses, can cause a disturbance in melatonin production.

4. **Alcohol:** Alcohol is a form of possession that takes control of peoples' bodies. Its function opens the vessel of the body and allows spirits to take over. The term "alcohol" comes from the Arabic word "al-kuhl," which means "body-eating spirit." The molecular alchemy of alcohol separates an object's essence from its physical form. The same way that drinking alcohol can separate the soul and essence of a person from their physical body.

5. **Pesticides:** Pesticides are a poison that impairs cognitive function and raises the risk of mental disorders.

6. **EMFs:** EMFs damage the pineal gland because they disturb electromagnetic fields. It has been demonstrated that shungite stones can protect us from electromagnetic fields (EMFs).

7. **Overall Lifestyle:** Living a poor lifestyle regulates the third-eye function and un-balances chakras. This includes: eating poorly, laziness, drugs, smoking, not enough exercise, not getting enough sleep, alcohol, watching porn, sex addictions, overspending, negativity, violence, overspending, and etc.

Conscious Earth

Vibrating energy fields are the means by which we communicate with the Earth, a living, sentient being. Plants and their natural environments are more capable of seeing and reacting to a multitude of environmental conditions than humans are. Plants are able to communicate with one another both above and below ground, and they have active social lives. All living things, including microbes, plants, and animals, are aware of environmental changes and adapt by changing their behavior. In order to increase survival, these behavioral modifications are based on adaptive and natural selection. Like humans, all other living things are conscious.

Plants have very complex systems that enable them to do incredible things, despite the fact that they are unable to think and act like humans. They function according to universal scales and rhythm. Time-sensitive genes in plants help them determine when to stop growing. The circadian rhythm, a 24-hour "body-clock," is present in both plants and animals. Plants can also experience stress from other activities and the environment.

Without a mind or a brain, they communicate extensively with each other and with insects in an effort to thrive and grow. They have functions just like nervous systems. Nature and plants also have memory since they can recognise and respond to different weather patterns. There are up to 15-20 distinct senses that plants possess, including human-like abilities to smell, taste, see, touch, and hear.

In 1966, polygraph expert Cleve Backster, who had previously worked for the CIA, tested the theory and discovered that the plants behaved differently depending on whether thoughts were positive or negative. Backster's team connected plants to polygraph machines and found that when a plant watched someone trampling on another plant, thereby killing it, it could recognise a "killer" from a lineup. It enrolled in a flood of electrical action. He then proceeded to find plants communicating telepathically. Plenty of studies since then continue to support the existence of conscious nature on our Earth.

Plants interact with one another in a variety of ways, and one of the closest things we have to telepathic communication is the "nanomechanical oscillations" vibrations that occur on the smallest atomic or molecular size. Plants also "bio-chat" by releasing tiny quantities of certain chemicals into the soil through their roots. This is known as the "rhizosphere" in biology. Every other living organism in the "root zone" receives signals from these substances, which are referred to as "root exudates."

But what happened to our relationship with nature? As conscious beings, why have we become so distant from our innate divinity? Everywhere you look, the Earth is living consciousness! Like humans and animals, plants are sensitive to their environment. As the Earth becomes more illuminated by light, many are also becoming more aware. The realm of consciousness encompasses more than just humans. In point of fact, all life, to some degree or another, is conscious.

The many different plants that grow in gardens and fields, the rocks we sit on, the soil we feel under our feet, the trees that cover the Earth, the sand that covers the beaches, oceans, lakes, and streams, are conscious in a sense of awareness that involves knowing itself to be alive to some extent. Therefore, whether we're talking about a tree, a rock, or a human, we may assume that all of them have some sort of feeling, no matter how basic or vague. When we treat nature with the highest respect, love, and care, we draw positive vibrations in return, resulting in a deliberate exchange of love and light. Nature is a powerful, lovable, and life-giving healer. When we observe the beauty of blossoms, trees, and flowers with minimal effort, we experience healing in numerous ways. Nature is electromagnetic, can feel, communicate, and is sentient, bringing us closer to this divinity and making it simple for us to raise our vibrations. Considering nature is the basis of our economy, society, and even our very life, we must realize that it must be treated with the utmost regard.

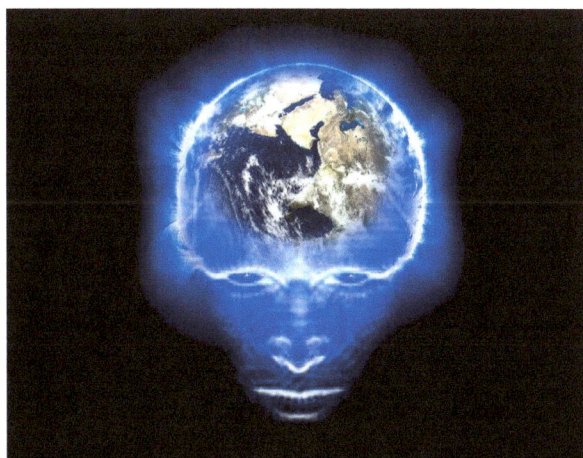

The Chosen Ones

A group of people who are a part of the savior's journey are the chosen ones. Those who work toward the goal of establishing a new earthly kingdom for the greater good. They are entirely people whose purpose is to aid in the preservation of humanity and raise the frequency and vibration of the planet. The chosen ones are old souls who have returned to Earth for a specific soul purpose, such as to bring about enlightenment or to complete a universal mission.

Others refer to them as "God's work" or "God's chosen" because they enter the darkest tribulations and shine light on it, until it is revealed. A lot of people are assigned missions, but only a few are chosen! In a planet we are losing, it is a small group of thousands attempting to continuously awaken large groups, occupying millions to billions. The average person today is allergic to wisdom and careless about the harm that continues to be done to Mother Nature, and this is the Earth we currently inhabit. In the hope that things will improve, the chosen ones take on the task of resolving this never-ending evil—a task that almost seems impossible but requires a big heart to bear all the suffering. In their attempts to solve a broken system and a damaged society, the chosen ones endure a lot. They put so much love and work into their mission, nevertheless, all they seem to receive in return is anguish and pain. The cost of being chosen is that they will always face a lot of obstacles. Most people think of chosen ones as helpless saviors who can't save themselves, and crazy people who don't know what they're saying. However, in actuality, the majority of the chosen ones are beyond their years and spiritually advanced.

Pain and suffering are a part of your destiny if you are chosen and now you have a very important mission to complete here on Earth. You can't back out now! You must keep up with this fight, the enemy knows and sees that! There's really a spiritual battle taking place. Are you currently sleepwalking or awakening?

The Christian bible refers to the group number of anointed ones as 144,000 people who are called the servants of God in Rev. 7:3 and God's redeemed people. When you put this into a spiritual perspective, 144,000 people are the anointed ones who have been sent to Earth to work as lightworkers and enlighten others; they are the leaders of the new kingdom.

Each and every individual has soul missions for the varied tasks and purposes here on this Earth, whether universal tasks, family-oriented, or for your community. If you carry this light and wake up, you will realize that people are still programmed and designed to work against you.

Those Born Awakened

Most people who are awakened from birth feel like "aliens" or "weirdos," and they don't really fit in with society. People who think outside the box and are critical thinkers couldn't care less about being 100 percent politically correct all the time. Most of the time, their parents misunderstand them and give them different labels. They are the ones who grow up thinking that there's something wrong with their personality or something off and strange about this planet. These are the awakened, and when they discover their spiritual path—which they eventually do—they transform into beacons of light for those in their environment. People who are born awake are frequently mocked, bullied, or ostracized for being different from other people or having different beliefs. They are frequently the target of gangstalking systems, which have been in place since birth and are designed to eliminate chosen ones off the face of this planet. The matter of fact is, the ones who are born with this light, are targeted by an enemy. Evil ones that will consciously place barriers in your way to slow you down. Negative spirits in the spiritual world will oppose the success of your divine purpose. They will block your path so that you cannot reach your goal. Furthermore, this is a light that is seen from birth!

Other Key Signs of a Chosen One

1. Presence, you stand out due to differences, such as talent, looks, energy, charisma, etc
2. Gang stalking, you've been targeted from birth or early on (for reasons like resentment, jealousy, wisdom, etc.)
3. You are seen as an outsider or a black sheep because of your unique thinking, perspectives, or critical problem-solving skills. People never understand you.
4. People stare at you in strange ways and patterns, which indicates that you have a powerful aura of light energy.
5. You pose a threat to all evil. They have their eyes on you and are aware of your potential.

6. Forced to walk the path alone. Everything you've accomplished is attributable to the difficulties and challenges you've faced on your journey on your own with little assistance.

7. If you are the only one in your family who has awakened or if you are genuine and come from a troubled or toxic family. Many angels come from demonic families.

8. Having the ability to fix, change, and provide others with valuable insight.

9. Typically quiet and reserved by nature.

10. You are singled out, people pick on you, or you naturally attract people.

11. If you can see what others cannot and come up with thoughtful and creative ideas.

12. Your soul is pure, compassionate, loving, and caring. You enjoy helping others and look forward to doing so.

13. Natural intelligence, coming from awareness, life, and critical thinking. (not from formal education)

14. A person who has always been in touch with the divine, the spiritual world, and wisdom and questioned everything in life.

15. An outsider. If you have always followed your own instincts and actions rather than those of others.

16. You never fit in with anybody, you are one of a kind, and learn to adapt and reason with anyone.

17. Innate ability to detect the emotional and energetic state of others (empathetic).

18. Lonewolf, a path you go down by YOURSELF.

19. If you've always felt alienated and different from other people.

20. If you've come to the realization that you have a higher calling after having a near-death experience (reminder to serve a purpose).

21. You innerstand you have a higher purpose, mission, and responsibility for the world since a young age or time of reason

Why Angels Are Born in Demonic Families

Angels are light, love, and full pureful energy but are seemingly born into demonic broken families. Angels are born into demonic families to break generational curses as a chosen one. They are the beings that will bring forth positive life and energy in a generational bloodline that is broken. Sometimes there are many children in the family, but there is that one child that has a message to serve or big success to achieve with their remarkable talent. Angels born into these families face a great deal of difficulty because they must overcome the challenges, ridicule, embarrassment, and total hardships of breaking through this family's pain and hard suffering. This cup is carried by the chosen ones, the angels! This is the very thing holy messengers came here to do, although it is difficult. Being raised in a dysfunctional household will prepare you for dealing with all the evil spirits, dark energy, and people you will encounter while on your journey. For some to take on this task, is a good thing, nevertheless, everything happens for a reason. In this brutal world, if you have a pure heart, you will face hostility. Therefore you must be grateful for the people who have contributed to your strength. Some souls opt to be born in more fortunate positions in order to take on tasks that will ease their path or enter a possibility for greater completion. Regardless of the path, it is all done for a greater goal for good. The intention is to shed light on crucial circumstances, and it is for this reason that angels are born into demonic families, to change and fixate on this destiny. Everyday there is no time to stop on this heavenly mission, so get back out there, angels, and complete your task because you have a purpose. Share your light and knowledge with the rest of the world!

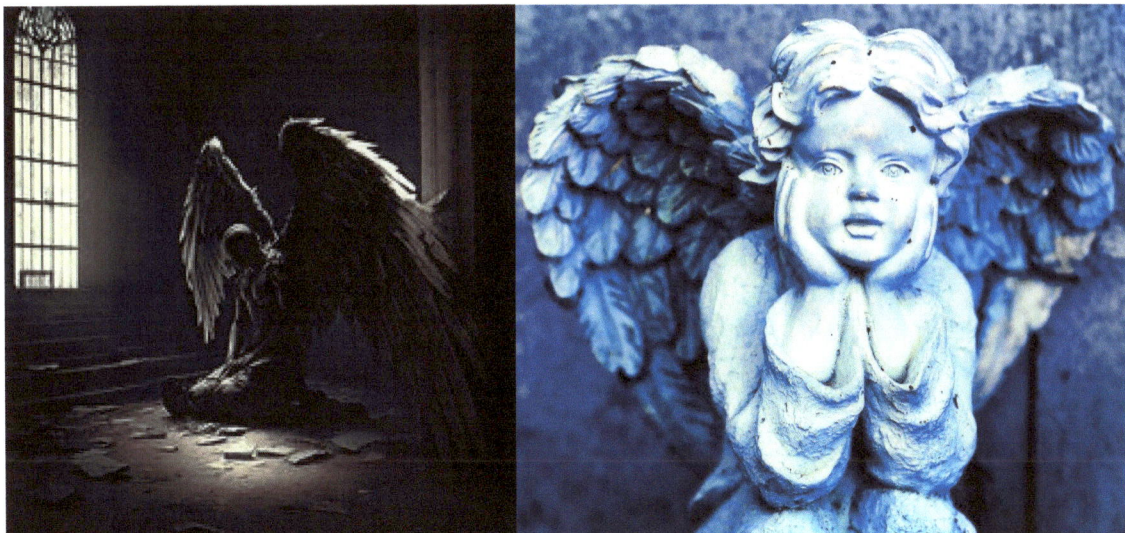

How To Find Your Soul Purpose

Finding your purpose is one of the most important things to understand about yourself while searching within. Many battle to track down the core of themselves and the internal qualities inside, because of this matrix infrastructure. The following are the key things to look for when searching within:

1. **Life Path Number:** Each life path number is unique and leads to ultimate soul fulfillment. It indicates part of your purpose of being on this Earth and your mission. In numerology, it is ultimately the essence of who you are. The life path number is similar to your Sun sign in astrology and suggests your strengths, identity, weaknesses, talents, and purpose. You will be intrigued to see the amount of connections and accuracy in your number as you discover more about it. The method is to take the numerical value of your date of birth, put all the digits together per category (year, month, day), and add it until you are left with a single digit. You may also just use a simple "life path number calculator" online to automatically calculate it for you.

2. **Natal Chart:** Your placements in signs, planets, and other astrological elements are determined by your birth chart. Each of us was given a magical birth chart that tells us who we are astrologically. Calculating the astrological aspects and delicate angles of your birth is done with a natal chart, which reveals our fundamental identity, our genesis. A natal chart can reveal a lot about your personality, motivations, and goals. All of these pieces of information help you learn more about yourself, accept who you are, gain insight, and appreciate the magical traits and characteristics you possess. Astrology is the path to self-discovery, where you learn to accept the things you can't change and understand why you're the way you are and adapt to the patterns you see.

3. **Blood Type:** Your blood type can determine the Starseed family you belong to. Some rare blood types are very important to royal lineages or have ties to star seed families from other planets. Your unique qualities may be identified based on your blood type, which is a direct result of your DNA and ancient ascended masters. It is the foundation of your bloodline.

- Starseeds are individuals that originally came from another planet and then reincarnated on Earth. A considerable lot of these people all have and spread an inborn reason for raising the vibration and consciousness of the planet, truth-seeking, and sharing their information and talents with the world. Since the dawn of human civilization, several extraterrestrial species have visited Earth and interbred with humans, giving each of us unique gene pools and lineages. This revelation can be comprehended gradually over time, through a series of discoveries or suddenly and greatly through an awakening of consciousness. Some of the awakened ones retain memories of their past, place of origin, and missions.

4. **Family Background:** The fate of your soul may be determined by your upbringing. Family backgrounds help you know what needs to be healed within your family and what is chosen to do out of it. Researching your family's history might help you learn more about earlier generations that you may not have known of. As a result, you develop a sense of personal identification and come to appreciate your culture and knowledge of your ancestry. It opens your eyes to your uniqueness.

5. **Meditation/Dreams:** Your meditation can assist you in communicating with your ancestors and locating inner guidance. Additionally, your dreams are a gateway to the astral planes, which could reveal parts of yourself and past incarnations.

6. **Starseed Families and Characteristics:** Raise the question of whether your soul came from Earth, or from extraterrestrial origins. If you've ever glanced up at the night sky and felt a connection with a brilliant planet or blazing cluster of stars, it is possible that your soul has a connection to a past existence. It is worthwhile to investigate a number of extraterrestrial families and races that have been documented throughout history.

7. **Specific Purpose:** What skills do you possess and what can you contribute to society, family, or your community? We are all present on Earth for a reason, one way or another. What goals do you have for yourself? Some of them are here to educate, raise the vibration of the planet, awaken family or friends, change lives, heal others, end family curses, provide valuable services, reach a higher self, clear karmic debt, and so on.

- Some people reincarnate on Earth after repeatedly failing to reach 5D (light), while others arrive as old souls to bring forth light and change this planet's dimensional polarity. Each of us has karmic debt and certain soul contracts that must be completed. The lists that follow—which I discussed earlier—will assist you in discovering your soul's purpose.

8. **Angel Numbers:** Angel numbers are signs that assist you in following your path and accomplishing your goals. They originate from the divine source; your higher self and your spirit guides.

9. **Other personal experiences, signs, and visions:**

- What signs, stages, and experiences, whether spiritual or physical, have you had to go through in your life?

- What visions and messages do you receive from your dreams or meditations?

- What personal goals and destinies do you have?

- What synchronicities do you experience?

- Are you one of the chosen? If yes, have you ever been a target in your life? Or, what indications can you use to confirm your experiences or mission?

- In general, what can you learn about yourself from all of your experiences, personal history, traits, signs, clues, visions, dreams, and goals? Combine them, do the inner work, and connect the dots.

- You will soon begin to realize the power and potential you possess within yourself as you evolve and begin your journey of inner work and soul-searching.

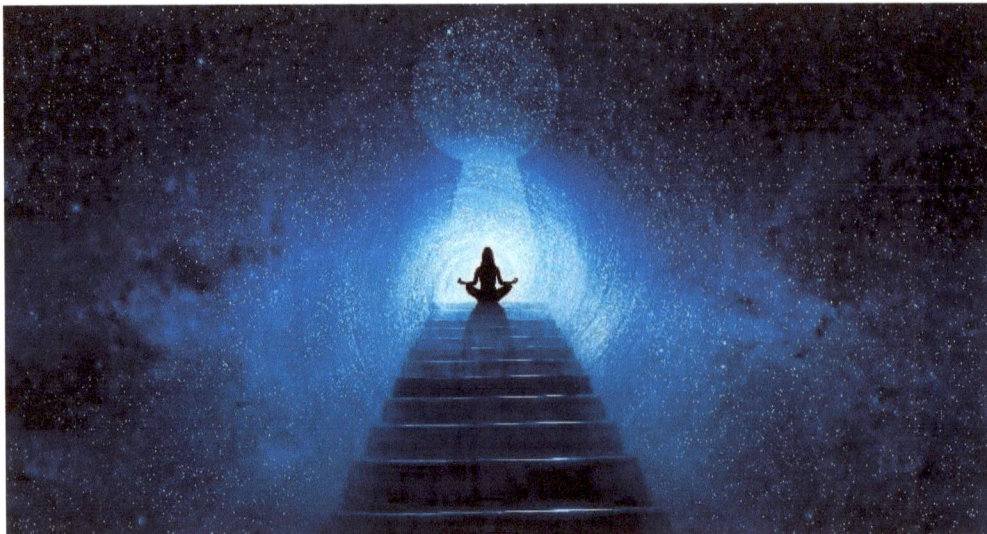

What Are We Made Out Of?

According to natural and scientific analysis, every part of our body originated in a star. In the earliest of times, simply the lightest of components existed which are elements like hydrogen, helium and minute measures of lithium. Through this course of generational turns of events, various stars have contributed to the components we find in our own planetary groups and those found inside us. Over multiple star lifetimes and billions of years, the majority of our human makeup is formed in stars which scientists have demonstrated and tested. Humans share 97% of the atoms and elements that make up life in our galaxy. This further demonstrates how the universe and all components of nature are inside each and everybody. Because we are composed of the elements that give life to galaxies, we are one with creation! The type of stars is a course of our cosmic development and addresses a basic impression of ourselves. We transcend flesh and blood as infinite beings of light!

For millennia, man has looked at the stars and considered what they are. We have made up stories and legends about them. One of these myths held that the stars were spirits or souls looking down on Earth. For instance, many of the constellations in Greek mythology were heroes who were given their places because of their heroic deeds. Second, if a decent life is lived, every soul has a companion star to which it returns to after death, according to Plato's Cosmology.

Stars are the souls of the universe; they are the places where our souls were created and where we will be watched in the afterlife. Stars, in my view, are merely portals, symbolizing the purgatory state in which our souls enter another realm or existence. I call them the afterlife's dwelling stages. The association between near-death experiences and stars is a surprising one. Near-death experiences (NDEs) often involve looking down into the human body and seeing a bright light.

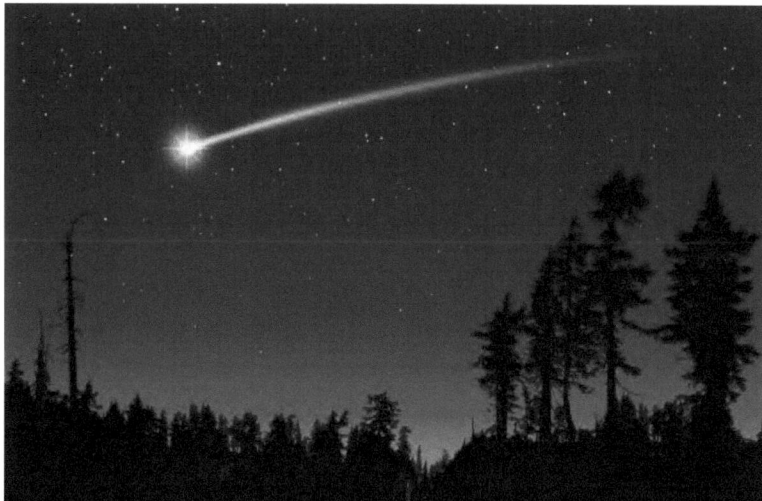

A Guide to Astral Projection - More To Life

The term "astral projection" is used to refer to a projected out-of-body experience (OBE) through which consciousness can function independently from the physical body and move around the astral plane. As someone with several astral projection experiences, I will simply provide the process of how to astral project and enter the spiritual realm.

Note: You must have already mastered meditation in order to perform astral projection

Preparation

1. **You must have a light body:** The light body is an astral body that connects to various bio-magnetic fields and body mechanisms which work within the etheric self. **To have this includes the following:**
- Raised Vibration: Fully raised vibration and positive/healthy mental state.
- Fasted: Fully fasted and cleansed, this includes non-toxic meals, GMOs, and a well-fasted state or empty stomach.
- Meditation: Meditation will bring you into stillness, clarity, and heightened consciousness.
- Be Clear: Addiction and dishonesty are drawbacks to this line of work. Holding clarity in your thoughts, will, and intention is important.
2. **Be in the right care and vibration:** Positive vibrations are necessary for positive experiences. Negative vibrations and well-being can result in unpleasant experiences such as spiritual attacks, fear, anxiety, and even possession.
3. **Must have positive energy and cleansing within you and around:** If you are afraid, you should not try this. Spirits can try to take advantage of your vulnerability. To get rid of bad spirits and energy, your environment must also be cleansed and clear. Uses of sages and candles can be suggested to clear the environment.
4. **Create The Right Environment and Atmosphere:** It is advised to try these techniques alone and in an isolated setting to avoid disturbances.

5. **Your consciousness must be awake:** Not right before sleep, typically during the morning or afternoon when you are awake.

6. **Astral Projection Hertz:** Prior to leaving the body, astral projection hertz can help put the body to sleep and stimulate the pineal gland.

Beginning: The goal is to make your physical body fall asleep, while your consciousness is awake, in order to travel outside of the body. You will travel with the soul through the vehicle of the pineal gland.

1. **Lay Down:** Lay down straight directly on the back in a vertical position to fully allow the soul to travel out of the body.

2. **Don't Move and Relax:** Do not move your body, lay down still and do not make any movements. You want to make your physical body go to sleep while keeping the mind awake.

3. **Close Eyes:** Close your eyes (let thoughts flow - begin mediation)

4. **Breathe In and Out:** Focus on breathing (hold breath every 2-3 seconds)

5. **Bliss State:** After 20m + you will reach the bliss state (hypnosis) you will now begin the mindfulness of moving the soul from the body. This stage is regularly known as the hypnagogic state. Relax your body to drift it off to sleep, but KEEP your mind AWAKE!

6. **Visualize 1:** Visualize your toes curling and uncurling, or your fingers clenching and unclenching, until it seems as though they are physically moving. Also, visualize your body flexing, but not literally.

7. **Visualize 2:** Enhance your focus to the rest of your body. Move your legs, your arms, and your head using only your imagination. Focus on imagining your body moving once at a time until you're able to move your whole body in your mind alone.

8. **Visualize 3:** Imagine yourself leaving your physical body using the rope technique. Envision a rope while laying down, and use the rope to climb out of your body. The consciousness will manifest and project these visualizations in order for this to work.

9. **Vibrations and Shaking:** You will presently feel your body shaking or begin to sweat. The waves and vibrations will begin to intensify at various frequencies. This is how your soul gets prepared to leave the body.

10. **Don't Panic:** When you reach this point, don't be afraid; just keep going until you give into the body's vibrations and trembling. Eventually, let the process flow and you will begin to emerge out of your physical body.

11. **Escape Physical Body:** Use your soul to move out of your body. If you try to physically move your body and you can't, your soul has successfully left the body.

12. **New Plane of Existence:** You will then first see pitch black, to multiple colors, and after a full 3rd person view. You will currently start to enter another plane of existence with your soul. As a soul, you would typically be able to see your own physical body laying on the bed. You can then travel to different dimensions, through the realms of portals, orbs, and other things.

13. **Confirmation:** Check to see whether your body is still there, look around the room and then depart. Investigate deeper.

14. **Explore:** Do not interact with any harmful entities while you navigate around. You'll always be able to return to your own body.

15. **Silver Cord:** An invisible cord keeps your soul always connected to your body, which is sometimes called a "silver cord." Your soul will be led back to your body by the force.

16. **Final:** Enter your physical body back again.

The Silver Cord: You won't suffer harm unless you believe it will. During OBEs, some people spend a lot of time outside of their bodies, which is believed to weaken the silver cord. The silver cord, however, cannot be weakened. Astral travel is strong, natural, and healing, so you shouldn't be concerned about it. Pure energy cannot be destroyed; it can only be transferred from one form to another. Although the silver cord cannot be cut off, if your soul is away from your physical body for a long period of time, it may take longer to return. However, the soul will always come back to the body since your spirit and body are connected.

Before attempting an astral projection, you run the greatest risk if you do not ensure that you are grounded in some way. To succeed at this, you must be prepared and in the right frame of mind. Not in a state of fear. Fearful behaviors in the astral realm can result in harm to the physical world. It can translate to scars, curses, bad luck, and spiritual attacks. It can take several tries to do this practice successfully. Astral projection provided me with a lot of my personal experiences and knowledge about the spirit world and extraterrestrials. It's an excellent way to discover things outside of the physical world.

How To Access The Akashic Records

The collective consciousness of all living things throughout history can be found in the Akashic Records. It can include your karmic debt, hidden parts of yourself, and past lives. It can be accessed by entering the mental plane of consciousness, which is linked to your own DNA and holds genetic memories. Only astral projection is allowed for direct access to the Akashic Records. Although your birthmarks, dreams, meditation, or family history may have previously given you some indications. Each experience will assist you in uncovering important things as well as deeply buried secrets within yourself.

FIRST STEP

1. **Questions:** You need to figure out why. For what purpose are you doing this? You should have received some clues about some aspects of yourself that you identified at this point.
2. **Make a List:** Make a list of all the specific information you'd like to have or access to. Make sure your inquiries are detailed.
3. **Ask Questions:** Ask questions about things you are unsure of and which you may already have some clues too. You can also ask questions about your personal life that can be helpful. Record them on paper.
4. **Considerations:** Consider just one concern at a time. The answers might not be obvious right away and instead reveal themselves when the moment is ideal.

SECOND STEP

1. **Declare Goal:** Declare your goal or express your inquiry out loud and seek guidance. It is advised to attempt this as an affirmation in front of a mirror once you are in the precise condition that you are aiming for.

2. **Begin Astral Projection:** To begin entering the altered state of consciousness (astral projection or meditation), locate a quiet location. At the same time you can ask for security; "Please shield me with light and protection as I begin my search, dear spirit guides, angels, or the universe (however you wish to say)."

3. **Ask Questions Prior:** When you've entered the meditative or bliss state, use your mind to ask; "to be granted access to the Akashic records."

4. **Enter Astral Travel Successfully:** Method of a rope or door portal: Most of the time, astral projection involves going through a door portal or a rope.

5. **Await for Information:** Wait for any signals or other information of any kind to enter your consciousness.

6. **Perceive Information:** The information can appear in a variety of ways. You might hear, see, taste, feel, or even smell something that may be intended to pass a message on to you.

7. **Contact:** Introduce yourself to what you've encountered and continue what you've contacted.

8. **Reflection:** After that, you can think about it and go back to the process if you want to, or even write down your experiences.

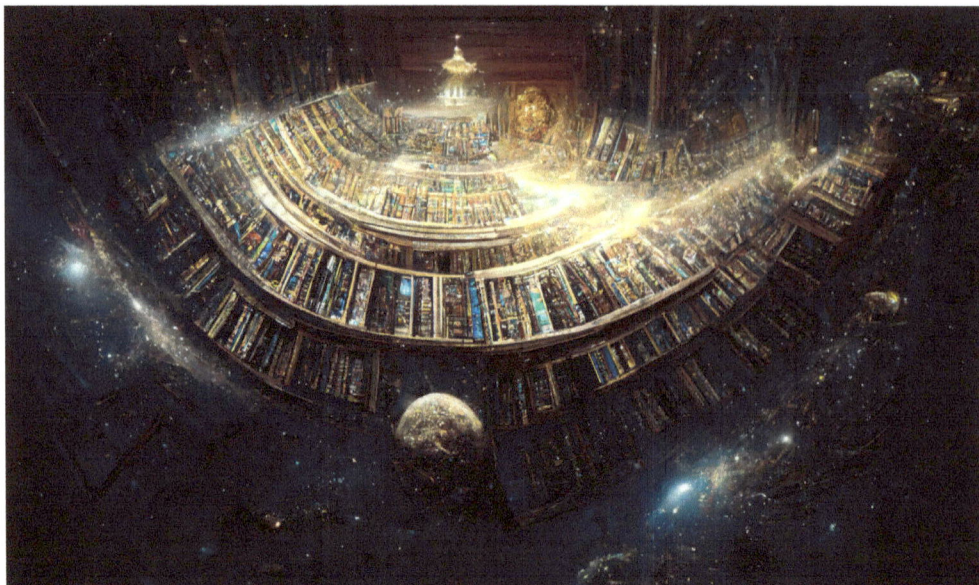

Sacred Sexuality The Elites Manipulation of Sexual Energy

The Sacred Number 6 and Numerology

The number six is associated with materialism, money, and worldly concerns. Because of this, Christians often refer to the number six as the number of sin, and in Hebrew numerology, six was often regarded as an evil number. From the Christian point of view, God created man and beasts on the sixth day, and men were given six days to work. Although there is no number that is intrinsically bad, there is an imbalance when the vibration of six is overemphasized.

When you see the number six repeatedly (666) on clocks, number plates, and buildings, it serves as a reminder to focus your intentions on more spiritual areas rather than on materialistic wants. You are being advised to turn within and seek spiritual guidance more when you see sixes. Celebrities and politicians that frequently use the '666 hand sign' show their admiration for the notion that the number six stands for the mastery of material affairs. Thus, the number 666 symbolizes an effort to cut off the link to limitless love in order to focus only on worldly activities like sex, power, and riches. The linguistic resemblance between the terms sex and six has a purpose. XXX stands for 666. The word 'sex' comes from the Latin verb 'secare', which means to cut off or separate. When prioritized, sex, like the number 6, becomes a force of constraint rather than development.

The Body Is So Much More

Humans' sexual energy or sex drive, is the body's most powerful energy source. The sexual energy that we all possess is the inner life force that sustains our creativity, discipline, and strength. It is our magic's primary source for ultimate creativity.

An orgasm is more complex than a simple sensation of pleasure. When the nervous system is supercharged with sexual energy during an orgasm, the outcome is a short circuit and a harmful release of energy. Whenever vital centers burn out, people grow impotent or lose interest in sex. This explains why sex toys and pornography are becoming more and more popular nowadays, as well as the widespread usage of Viagra and other related drugs. It's all artificial pleasure. People start to have more extreme sexual obsessions since the areas that used to make them happy are no longer exciting. By placing an excessive amount of focus on the vibrations of six and limiting the revival of sacred sexuality, many people have become trapped in a vicious cycle.

What the general public is lured into nowadays is participating in sexual liberation, this is actually sex slavery. Sexual expression cannot be addressed by engaging in sex only for pleasure. Using that sexual energy in more inventive ways is the actual solution. Naturally, this requires discipline, but discipline for the sake of salvation rather than posing self-inflicted harm. As both boys and girls get closer to puberty, they have an increase of more sexual energy. However, since they have already been exposed to a destructive worldview, this energy is usually never fully explored correctly. Through advertisements and so-called entertainment, unbalanced views towards sex are promoted to us. It's very difficult to escape being exposed to this inverted sexual seduction often when we encounter so many sexualized bodies in the media.

Energy Extraction Matrix

Sexual energy is one of the key methods that this matrix is kept in place. The elite use our own sexual impulses to control and enslave us. They set up a control grid around us with images of inverted sexuality as part of a black magic pact to allow spirits to feed off of our energy. Then, to further reinforce this world built on fear and control, these demonic powers turn our sexual energy against us. Fear and suffering act as batteries that store our sexual energy. The matrix is a dreamworld created by machines that were created to keep humanity in check. The elite are using our children's latent sexual energy by abusing them in a systematic manner in order to transform them into this. Children are more vulnerable to this energy than adults because of the panic and suffering they experience during the act, which makes it more than that of adult sexual abuse. Pedophilia therefore plays a significant part in the energy extraction matrix that drives it. The narrative that most of you are familiar with is either Pizza Gate or Pedo Gate, although child abuse networks have been exposed for years by whistleblower after whistleblower.

It takes a fear-based energy to maintain a dark, false reality within the confines of this hologram. Fear is limited, whilst love is limitless. The power of love is halved when there is an emphasis on material things like sex, which when unbalanced leads to anxiety and a mentality based on limitation. Because of this, the misleading matrix that we now live in cannot be destroyed without love. It produces vibrations that are more stronger than fear ever could. Love is a force that can be used without needing to be restrained. Love already overcomes every form of fear that it encounters. Another reason inverted sexuality is common is that the elite needs us to be preoccupied.

The higher spiritual advantages of life are usually overlooked by those who spend their time pursuing sexual pleasure. Most importantly, the endless search for sexual fulfillment takes our focus away from the task at hand, which is acting as a conduit for truth. As a result, we can shift this reality's structure from a system of control to one of love. Lust is an insatiable force that energetically eats its practitioner. For instance, all forms of sexual energy abuse are connected to the delusions of wealth and power. As a male, I can assure you that many men are drawn to careers in politics, show business, and music, because they provide more opportunities for promiscuous sex and status.

Today's sexual attitudes are characterized by rampant sexual dominance, which is mostly expressed by males. Our attitudes towards sexuality are a reflection of the imbalance between feminine and masculine traits in our culture, which overemphasizes the values of the left brain. Tenderness and passion have also been lost in society's concept of sex, just as the dynamic of care (the basic concept of the divine feminine). Right now, we need the divine feminine principles to come back to life. It is now necessary to teach and rediscover the sacred component of sexuality that has been kept secret.

When a male loses his semen, an essential fluid, it is referred to as the "little death." The term "la petite mort," which describes a sexual climax, is typically translated as "the little death." The literal translation, however, is a momentary dilution or loss of awareness during ejaculation. Men lose vital minerals and nutrients as a result of semen. B6, B12, and E vitamins are among them. Additionally, major amounts of the minerals copper, calcium, magnesium, zinc, and selenium are lost. Frequent masturbation and ejaculation overstimulate the parasympathetic nervous system, which causes an overproduction of sex hormones and neurotransmitters including acetylcholine, dopamine, and serotonin. Due to this overproduction and stimulation, these chemicals actually become less abundant over time, just like we see with extensive drug use. Vitamins are vital, but the seminal fluid has a far higher energy capacity. Men who lose this fluid suffer a loss that impairs creativity and self-control.

Sacred Sexuality

Most people use their phones or computers to watch porn while masturbating. When we browse the internet on our laptops and phones, which are black mirrors, we align with the vibrations of whatever information we are viewing or reading. Since pornographic websites are filled with sexual energy abuse and deviance, negative spirits can be produced through our black mirrors. Why do you think that free and accessible material like online porn exists? It keeps sexual distortions at high levels and enriches the elites since it is a tool and weapon utilized for their benefit. In pornography, the human body is often seen as a tool for pursuing personal pleasure. Particularly, both men and women are impacted by humiliation.

Watching most porn is a black magic ritual because it concentrates energy on twisted sexuality. As a result, watching two people engage in open sexual activity while you observe this energy exchange is equivalent to a ritual. Similar to watching porn, when candidates for a ritual perform an energy exchange, others watch. When you masturbate while watching porn, entities and demons always leach sexual energy from you, opening doors for portals and demons to participate in the ritual as well. Our genitals are actual real-life portals that can generate life and bring forth new energy. However, when used irrationally we become a complete waste, filled with negative effects energy drawn into us. If we want to enter a new paradigm in which our sacred nature is reignited, we must focus on producing that sacredness in the area of sexuality since our concentration is a vehicle for creation.

Numerous mental illnesses and conditions, including depression, anxiety, exhaustion, loneliness, mood swings, a negative body image, brain fog, reduced memory, psychosis, and other factors have been linked to pornography. People are willing to give away their most powerful energy to random people on pixelated screens like slaves, in order to create the illusion of a few brief minutes of pleasure.

Hollywood has totally diminished the term "semen" into "nut," to declassify the importance of sacral and astral energy. These terms were used to decrease or minimize the importance of a source of energy that is essential to our bodies. Media and entertainment regularly promote this catchphrase since they profit from it. The mainstream media teaches us that watching porn or masturbating, which are both unnatural and harmful behaviors, are beneficial. This is another matrix attack on society by leading people to feel that what is good for them is actually bad. In order to get people to repeat the same act of wastefulness and degeneracy, advertisements and commercials will continue to push sexual material online.

The same factors apply to women; pornographic viewing and masturbation weaken the root, solar plexus, and heart chakras, while also exchanging energy with other spirits and demons present in the space. We need to learn how to control our urges and make smarter use of our energy. Even though the majority of women do not ejaculate, they should still protect their vital life energy. The bottom half of the body continues to be the dominating locus for the discharge of female sexual energy. During sex, more energy is released, from men, the masculine sexuality. The receptive nature of feminine sexuality, however, absorbs energy in. Because they are absorbing vital fluid, it is essential that women are aware of the sexual exchange. Sex is always an exchange of energy, and both men and women share what they have. So basically in the event that a female or male that doesn't take care of themselves, is vibrating low, or has unhealed trauma imparted inside them, that energy is then shared with one another and, even passed on to other people. These negative effects will reflect in their reality, whether they realize it or not.

When women acquire an addiction to picking up this release, we categorize them as promiscuous. Instead of just being interested in sex, sexually promiscuous women are unaware addicts to this release and absorption. Instead of learning how to channel their own sexual energy and waiting to share it in the heart space of a loving partner, they absorb the energy of others with little to no genuine connection. This energy wave has shortcomings. It is an adrenaline rush that is felt both during and following intercourse. After that, it declines, which causes issues because the female fails to consider their partner's energy.

Just as it is unhealthy for men to carelessly release their own sexual fluids, taking sexual fluid by women is also dangerous. Sex involves not just the exchange of body fluids but also the exchange of auras. A part of our partner's energy goes into our aura during sex, while a bit of our own energy departs our aura and enters theirs. During sex, we create an energetic connection with our partner. Their thoughts, emotions, and desires leave imprints on our aura that, if not cleansed, may remain with us. Compared to sexually transmitted diseases, sexually transmitted entities are a much larger and more widespread problem.

Sexual Masculine Imperative

Men should relapse on sperm once every 64-74 days when sperm regenerates and replenishes at the end of the sperm cycle. This is typically the time when sperm that have been stored, come out and are replaced by new ones. It is advised for those in "monk mode" or on the "semen retention" journey to continue their streak of abstinence and balance their energy through the kundalini spine. Meditation, deep breathing, engaging in physical activity, and grounding, all work together to energize the entire body and store sexual energy in the appropriate places, like the spine/kundalini region. Regardless of the amount of sexual activities that men and women engage in, we should all balance and awaken our energy through our kundalini spine so that it can be created and powered throughout our entire energy vortexes. This will enable us to control sexual urges and cultivate energy for higher creativity.

The amount of times someone chooses to have sex is completely up to the person. However, it is important to know who you are sleeping with and what habits you are cultivating. Each and one should be aware and conscious of the spiritual and physical effects to cultivate a standard for themselves and best towards their own ability. If you don't have your own standard taking into account the negative consequences, then you are mindless and again a slave to your own ego.

Men who engage in sexual activity or ejaculate daily, (which is not advised for men) lose vital minerals and vitamins and have erratic energy depletion. The brain releases oxytocin, which increases arousal and excitement during sexual activity, once it wears off, some people may experience extreme exhaustion. If this is often occurring on several occasions or in a week you are actually wasting more energy than you think. Instead, conserve your energy for the tasks you wish to complete in your life and use it for meaningful purposes. The most important piece of advice I can provide is to avoid porn and masturbation. Masturbation and pornography viewing decrease your spiritual currency, weakens your aura and can have an adverse effect on your mental health.

Sexual Feminine Imperative

We are energetic beings, and during sexual activity, the energies of the partners mix. This is a foundation that never changes, and it is essential that everyone recognises this in order to have the awareness to take rational care of themselves without resorting to lust or ignorance.

Porn puts a standard for people to follow, even in terms of physical attractiveness. Such as the particularly ideal look of a slim thick body, curved hips, flawless skin, and pretty face. These norms are all deeply ingrained in pornography, modeling, and advertisements—all of which are designed to arouse sexual desire in viewers. Advertising is full of endless examples of women's hypersexuality. These are damaging perceptions that lead to insecurities, low self-esteem, unrealistic standards, jealousy, anxiety, depression, odd and abnormal fantasies, and stress. All of those harmful aspects of pornography result in warped views of sex and sexuality as well as distorted attitudes towards both men and women. Rewiring the brain is necessary to promote a reset in these distortions, and practicing continence can be a way for women to reset their perception of their own sexuality. Regardless of gender, the negative and spiritual effects of porn remain the same.

Birth control pills are being used more often today, which is impacting women's mental health, vibration, and frequency as a whole. A whole generation of women use birth control, which they thought would free them, but it actually made them more likely to have cancer, depression, and infertility. Birth control can raise the risk of liver and cervical cancer as well as the likelihood of breast cancer by up to 38%. These effects are overlooked by many. All vital minerals, including vitamin B9, vitamin B12, zinc, selenium, magnesium, and, most significantly, vitamin V6, are substantially reduced when birth control is used. This significantly raises the risk of developing multiple deficiencies. When using the pill, hormones are greatly altered, which makes one much more emotional and encourages impulsive and rash decision-making. On birth control, emotional intelligence—your capacity to comprehend and control your emotions—deteriorates significantly as well. Studies have demonstrated side effects like mood swings, depression, and anxiety, all of which have a significant impact on vibration. It causes one to lose all emotional control and puts them in a low, unbalanced state of energy, which hinders all of the chakras, from the root to the crown. People will live their lives however they choose to at the end of the day, yet maybe these facts can help some by putting certain things into perspective.

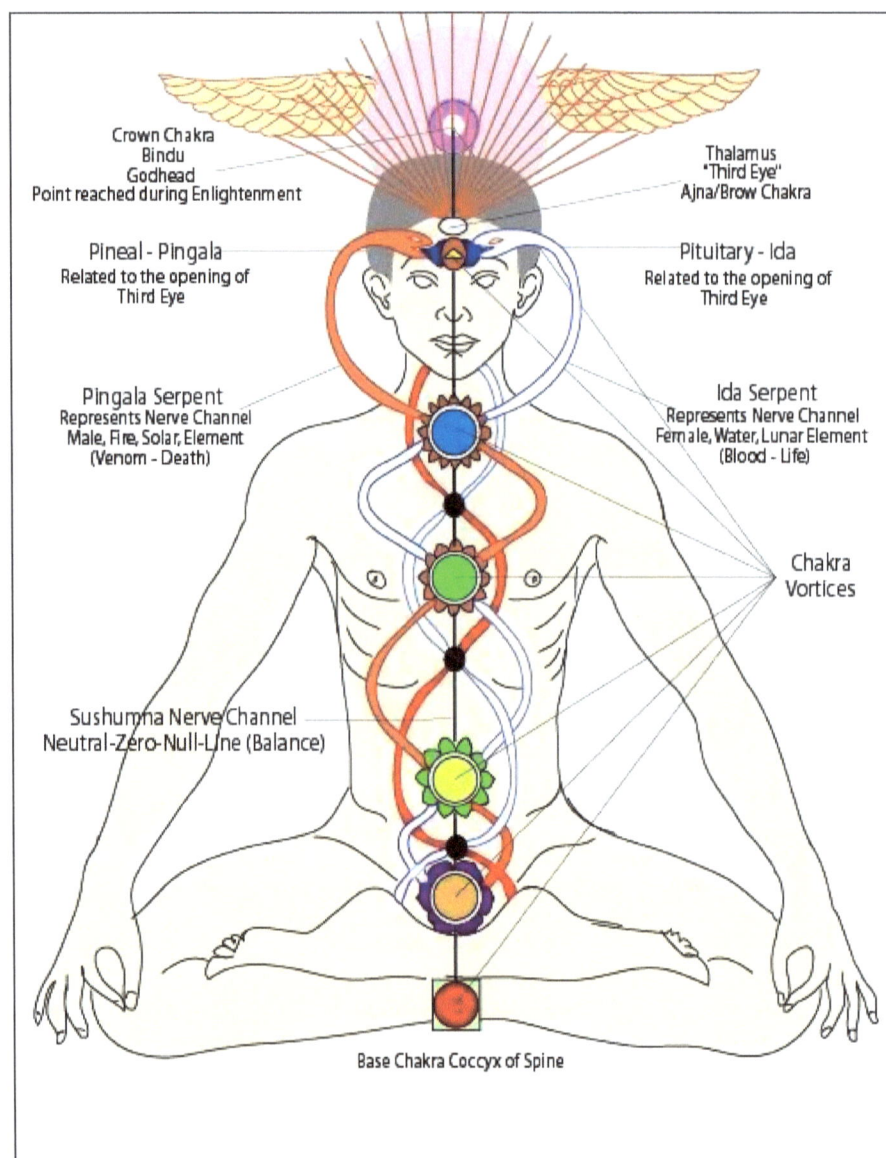

The Chest Is A Portal - Body Snatching

The human chest has the capacity to connect to different energy fields within its radius frequency since it has a subtle quantum attribute. The heart chakra region, which controls the rib cage, lungs, heart, circulation, skin, hands, arms, and upper back, is situated in the center of the chest.

Front   Back

The heart chakra is vulnerable on many different levels when it is weak. A weak heart chakra will attract and feed off of low energy and will be exposed to body snatching. Body snatching leaves a human vessel susceptible to uninvited spirits and demons. As your energy awareness increases, you can really see changes and feelings within your energy signature. The chest is where energy primarily travels and is held. For example, alcohol is a substance that makes you possessed when intoxicated.

A GALVANISED CORPSE

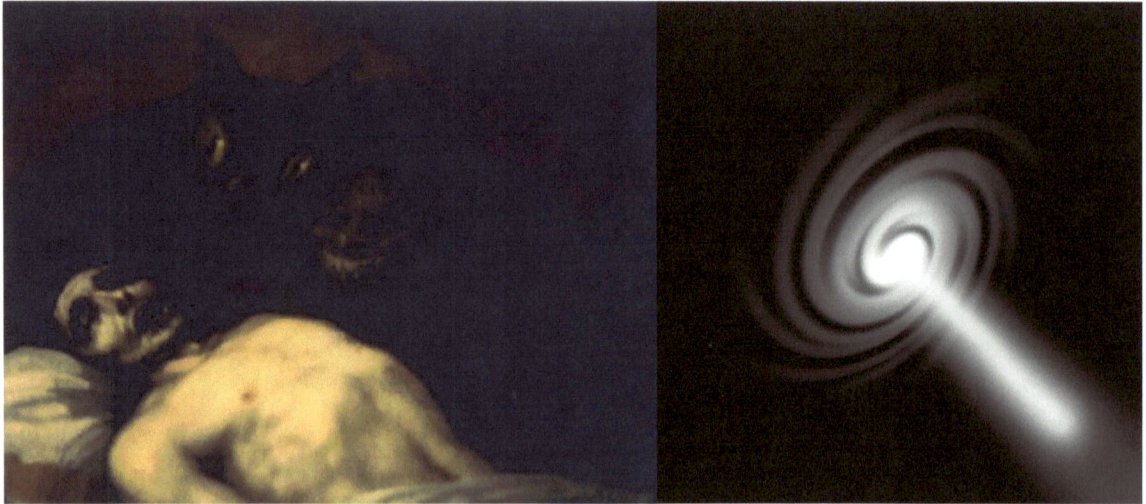

When the human body's frequency drops too low and its toxicity rises too high, the soul departs from the body and hovers around it. It makes the human body vulnerable to spirit attachments. An unbalanced system (chakras) leads to open spirits within energy vortexes (portals) within the human body.

Shadow Figures

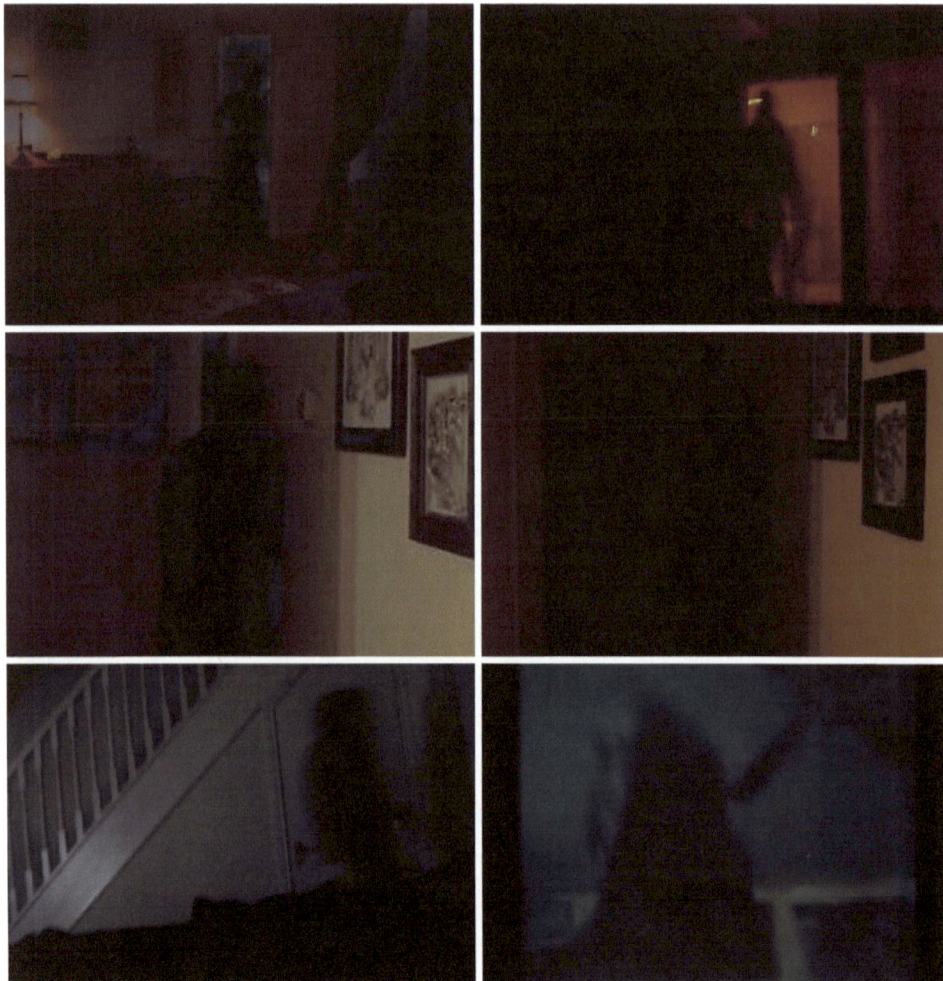

Have you ever wondered what that being was in the corner of your eye? Or what spirit you were seeing as a kid that was hovering over your bed? Or those brief moments where you see a spirit in your house but it disappears? Well, these are shadow figures, and it is identified with a phenomenon of spiritual beings in higher dimensions who dwell in the physical realm. Shadow figures are spiritual beings who travel to Earth to observe the human experience from a spiritual perspective. Many civilizations, religions, and belief systems consider them to be supernatural beings from the underworld. The Choctaw Nalusa Chito and the Islamic Jinn are two examples. The shadow figures are supernatural inhabitants of other realms and universes. It is commonly seen during "sleep paralysis," a situation in which the soul has halfway left the body. A person is awake but unable to move or talk when they wake up or fall asleep because their soul isn't in direct control. Sleep paralysis happens in 8–50% of people's experiences at one point in their life.

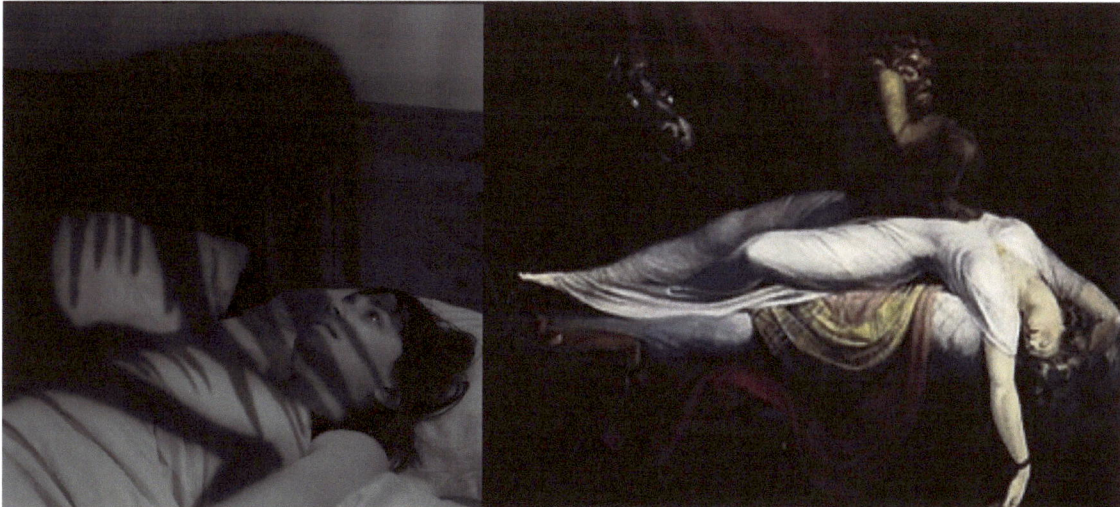

The auric field, which is collectively encompassed by a color or essence of an energy field, can be persisted by shadow figures. Due to their existence in other dimensions, people who have had other kinds of psychedelic experiences—in and out of body experiences—have reported seeing "shadow figures." Additionally, visual hallucinations are also mental representations that are produced as a result of various encounters and manifestations of extraterrestrial lifeforms. It is believed that shadow people are connected to alien life and are frequently "perceived" as an assembly of negative energy.

Reports about shadow figures are often negative. According to some accounts, shadow figures cast spells and curses, drain energy, instill fear, cause victims to have negative thoughts, and generally give victims an unforgettable experience. Shadow figures are able to body snatch in low vibrational vessels using a fear-based concept. Spirits with malicious purposes gain from making humans feel uneasy and frightened.

Paranormal Passions

Paranormal passions are where individuals tend to favor experiences in the dark spiritual realm. Examples can be seen of stories of women having sexual affairs with "ghosts," because they tend to bond more with spirits. These demonic spirits are known as succubus (female demon) and incubus (male demon), which appear in dreams to seduce a person to cause harm or drain their energy. These demons require vital sexual energy in order for them to survive.

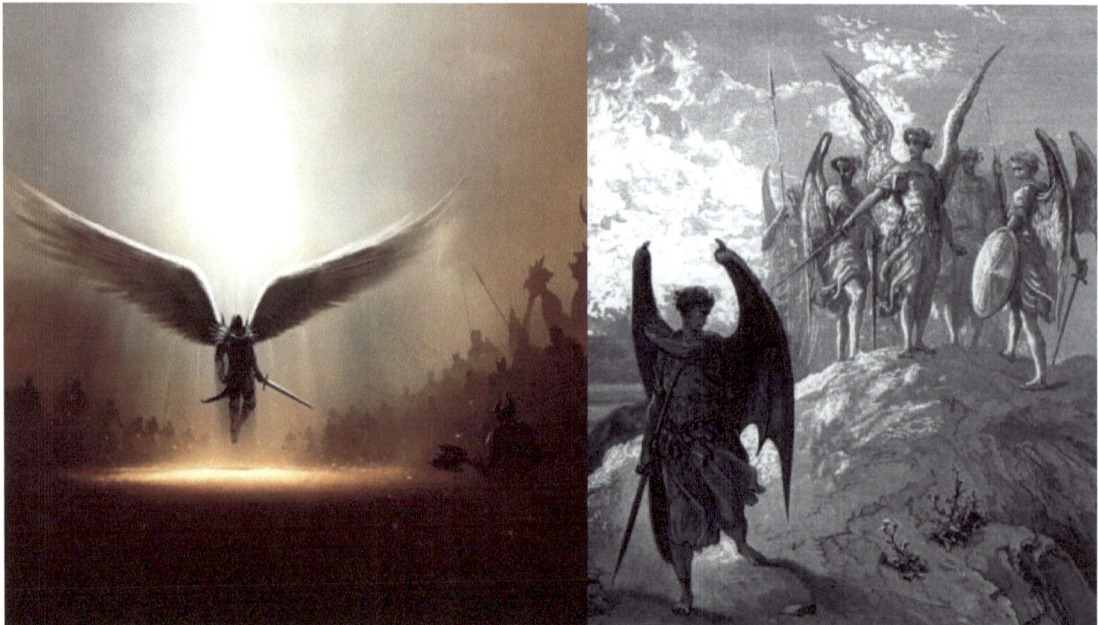

- A biblical reference is the watchers in the Book of Enoch. The watchers, or Iyrin in Aramaic, are angels sent to Earth to watch over humans in the Book of Enoch. At the behest of their leader Samyaza, they soon develop a lust for human women and defect to wrongfully teach and procreate with humans. Their offspring were hybrids of angels and humans and grew to enormous heights known as the Nephilim.

- The attraction to ghosts or the stimulation of one's sexuality by reflections in mirrors is a condition known as "Spectrophilia." This relates to the supposed phenomenon of sexual interactions between ghosts or other supernatural spirits and humans. Seduction and temptation are common themes in traditional ghost stories.

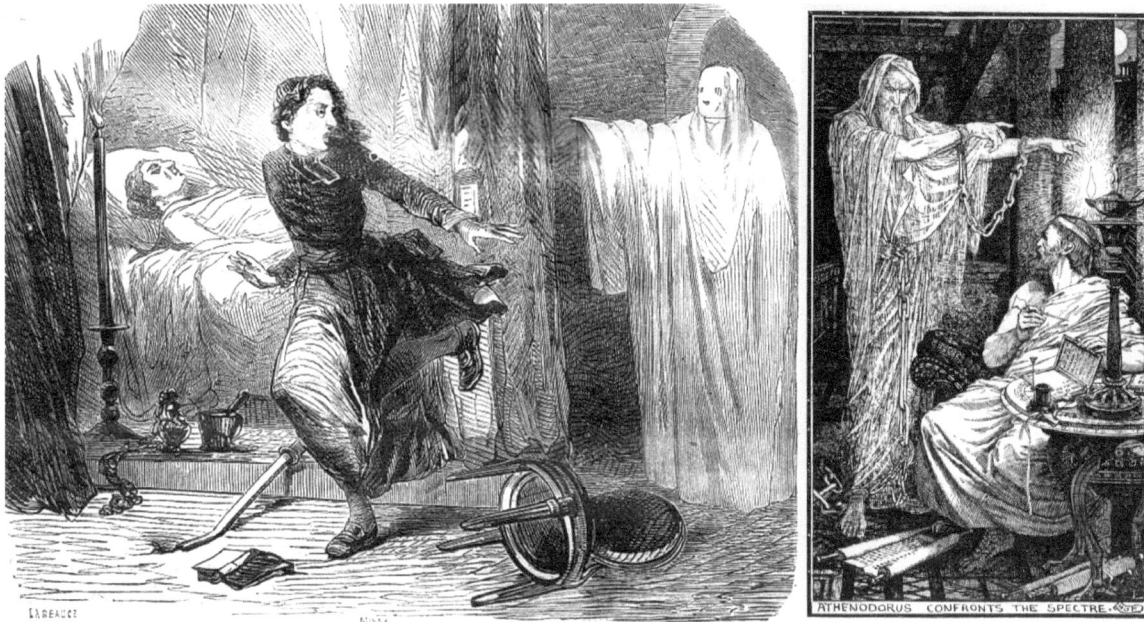

ATHENODORUS CONFRONTS THE SPECTRE.

My personal consensus following has led me to the conclusion that 25%, or one in four people, had experienced sexual experiences with supernatural beings. Few people who have had this experience develop a fixation or impulse to keep returning to a part of themselves that enables them to continue having sexual relations with spirits. As a result, people have fallen victim to these kinds of incidents and are possessed and controlled by these spirits. One of the side effects of having sexual encounters with spirits is having wet dreams. An incubus or a succubus will typically appear as a lover or crush and will force sexual impulses during the dream, which compels one to ejaculate. This enables the spirits to feed off that energy. When they succeed, they typically leave an impression on your subconscious and memory. The majority of experiences with paranormal sex almost feel like they are being held against their will or tricked by a lover to drain energy. They may appear as normal humans in dreams but have the ability to shapeshift and become hybrid beings/demons during sex. Similar to sleep paralysis, these experiences give the victims the impression that they are very real and that they are unable to move during the event.

Spiritless Humans / The Consciousness Split / Polar Opposites

Over the years I've always questioned why certain people seem very hollow and empty inside and why people are almost operating as if they are on autopilot. Well, I have gotten several emails and messages from people asking about the same thing and coming to this conclusion. This is an observation I had since I was a child, but as I suddenly grew older, I realized that society is being programmed to act like each and every individual instead of themselves. People try to catch up with the most recent trends or conform to and subscribe to the popular attitude and way of thinking that the mainstream media promotes. This aspect is hurting them from the inside out. Nowadays, there is less individualism and more copies, as a result of people mimicking each other's actions and personalities to fit in. Light and darkness, spirited and spiritless, soulful and soulless, awake and asleep, and so forth, are at odds with one another in our world. In these confines, there will always be this reality—an opposing force to everything.

Characteristics

Spiritless people tend to be materialistic and egotistical. These people can also share qualities such as being narcissistic or mundane, optimally being very dull and to themselves on a moral high ground. These traits through observation are levels through the social exterior, lack of individuality, critical thinking, and having a hard-headed mentality. Any other opinionated beliefs outside of the norm will sound crazy and outlandish, and lack comprehension of anything beyond the physical reality. They have no interest in such metaphysical matters except flashy clothes, accessories, or entertainment, to boost their social image. These individuals are sometimes referred to as "bots," which refers to those who have been programmed by 3D concepts and lack being personable. They also appear incapable of empathy, soul-searching, or questioning things beyond this physical reality. Empathy to them only appears when it's beneficial for them.

What else you can find is there is no spark or essence in their consciousness, whether they are intellectual or not. I tend to believe these people operate highly within their "R-Complex" or "Reptilian Brain," operating through animalistic and rudimentary views. As human beings, we should have some spark and difference behind us, but it only seems to remain for people who typically have a sense of their own beliefs, personality, and individualism. That's what brings someone's self out.

Missing Component

Something is missing, this goes beyond the physical factors. It is the soul, which calls to a higher component of consciousness which is absent in some people. The term "soulless" deals with someone completely devoid of feeling and of their own. They do have some kind of soul energy by being alive, but the soul is not imbued with a higher spark of true consciousness and self-awareness. Therefore the spark which I would like to call "spirit" is the individualized consciousness and traits which represent one's true self. In each incarnation, it gains knowledge and experience in order to develop further and reach its full potential. It is the divine god-spark, the source of free will, and the inner conscious observer that makes up this being.

Not every human has a spirit nor is connected within themselves. Therefore they have no self-awareness, individuality, wisdom, empathy, or conscience. Without spirit, they are temporary beings whose awareness forms shortly before birth and vanishes shortly after death. And if so, then for them, spiritual life lessons serve no purpose, karma from past lives does not exist, there is no higher self-acting as guidance, nor would they have a genuine interest in anything that serves a purpose beyond their current mortal existence. Therefore it is to be expected that they are particularly materialistic, and mundane in their ambitions; observation confirms this as well.

Other Missing Components

We communicate with the physical world through the body's biological interface. The body has its own genetic predispositions, biological urges, instincts, social programming, and behavioral patterns when it is born. These predetermined factors combine to give rise to an artificial intelligence that, by default, controls the body like an airplane's autopilot system. This artificial intelligence can further be known as the "ego." Its main goal is to optimize behavior for the physical and social environment around it in order to maintain the body's survival. To put it another way, external conditioning trains the ego to succeed in the conditions where it was formed. It is like an etheric computer hardware that simulates a living identity based on its environment. It serves as a mimicker, similar to something that can automate social interactions and serve as an identity mask. This function has been programmed from birth and operates in its immediate surroundings. Similar to a video game in that the characters have human-like appearances and behaviors, and when the player is not controlling them, they appear to operate autonomously. The spirit exists fully outside of linear time, while the ego is wholly a product of the past. Additionally, the spirit is an everlasting pairing of consciousness, whereas the ego is a characteristic of matter. The two are directly at odds with one another. Our everyday consciousness is a mixture of the two, but one can opt-in what proportions to work through the spirit or solely the ego.

Negatives of Lacking a Spirit

Think about what happens if a person lacks spirit but has a body, ego, and soul. Firstly, physical factors like genetics and environment would have the most impact on how they are. Their ego would be the source of their appearing intellect. And without the spirit as a tick, their ego would rule. As a result, in line with the ego's purpose, such individuals would be wholly devoted to their own survival (both material and social). Those with spirit who are aware of their spiritual urges often make conscious decisions that are contrary to their interests in the world of social, finance, or ego. They are able to succeed higher without having the constant battle between the urges of the ego.

Upon death, spiritless people face the same cycle over and over again. People who lack spirit cannot benefit spiritually from life's challenges, learn spiritual lessons, or pass on what they have learned to later incarnations. As a result, they are uninterested in learning lessons of humility, empathy, compassion, comprehension, or forgiveness. There cannot be real freewill or meaningful lessons to be learnt in the absence of spirit. The law of chance and the law of nature apply solely to the spiritless, who have no belief in karma. While a person with spirit may be born with karmic disadvantages, those without spirit would just have these disadvantages by accident or inheritance and they would not serve any higher metaphysical purpose. The same is true of when and how they die; unlike spirited people, who may have fluidly planned out their lives before incarnating, including how they will die. Spiritless people pass away at random and without meaning unless their passing plays a significant role in a spirited person's pre-incarnation script. Spiritless people almost serve as pawns for the matrix which is the physical representation of an AI player within the world.

Other elements that are still missing include synchronicities, higher intuitive guidance, significant symbolic dreams, and their own unique hand of fate. People without spirit don't go through any of these things since they can't or don't need to. A spiritless individual doesn't require such messages, because meaningful dreams primarily serve to alert a person to spiritual imbalances that need to be corrected. Without a stable core of personality, the "Higher Self," which is a perfected expression of spirit, cannot exist. Furthermore, they lack the inner intuitive guidance that may help them overcome life's obstacles in the absence of a Higher Self. In contrast, a spiritless person would pass away by accident whereas a spiritual person would experience strange synchronicities, signs, and messages to prevent them from an early death.

The spiritless do not require the higher chakras—the heart, crown, or third eye—because these are the only ones that connect to the spirit. They only connect to the lower ones, which deal with emotions, personal stability, and intellectual aspects which are present in everyone. They are unable to access the third eye, which allows for extra-sensory perception, or the heart, which is responsible for compassion and empathy. No matter how vibrant they appear to be on the surface, spiritless people are dull and lifeless on the inside because their etheric or auric vibrations lack specific colors and have a lower overall quality. Some people don't have any spirit, and as a result, their upper chakras are likewise absent. You will see how this concept explains the complete range of observations that exist on so-called "empty" people if you carefully consider what this involves.

Pawns of The Matrix / The Pawn Class

All people who are programmed by higher authority belong to the pawn class. They are completely spiritless artificially intelligent beings that have been programmed and conditioned. They are conditioned to act like everyone else through a variety of cues; in a sense, they are like background characters who play a role in the matrix's society, while those in higher authority consciously control the pawns. The pawn determines their appearance as well as their physical interactions with the environment, however, it is their consciousness and spirit that sets them aside from other beings.

Difference Between Spiritless and Spiritually Asleep People

People who are spiritually asleep are more like people who are born open-minded and able to access higher consciousness, but who become entangled in the matrix and ego, which prevents them from developing their spirituality. They may exhibit spirituality-related attributes, but a significant portion of them is still trapped in the limitations of the third dimension and materialism. People who are spiritually asleep may see synchronicities, messages from their dreams, or angel numbers, but they don't always take them seriously and end up doing the wrong thing. They may fall into the category of immaturity and still be subject to the repercussions of karmic debt caused by poor decisions. Some people lack spirit, while others are asleep to spirit. When a person is completely awakened and spirited, they are more vulnerable to future karmic damage than others, because they have already grown to understand the effects of their decisions.

Spiritless people lack potential completely, and cannot grow spiritually. This is not just a speculative assertion; rather, it is a lesson learned through dealing with too many of these people who, although receiving a lot of support and opportunities for change, never showed any sign of evolution or growth. They adjust, at best, but more as a result of conditioning rather than real understanding. Because they do not operate within those confines, they do not experience the same karmic debt, spiritual trials, or effects as spirited people. They lack certain aspects and comprehension that are associated with higher or spiritual rationality when making decisions.

The lifestyles of the spirited people are in line with their needs on a spiritual level. Thus, there is a correlation between their level of spiritual growth and lifestyle. Because they only require a basic existence, baby souls will lead crude lives. Anything more would be too much for them to handle or gain. The spiritless, on the other hand, live any life they are forced into by circumstance or their own cleverness. Whether it be as a beggar, corporate executive, or well-known novelist. The lives of the spiritless are not governed by any spiritual limits or guidelines since they lack any spiritual requirements. And because of this, "empty" individuals are not all simply spiritually dormant or undeveloped; rather, a group of people who, regardless of their way of life, social status, intellectual ability, or physical appearance, all share the same inertness behind their eyes.

Psychologists refer to the more severe cases of a lack of spirit as having psychopathic, sociopathic, or narcissistic personality disorders. Spirited individuals who meet this description are misled and captive to their egos, yet they are also rehabilitable. Instead of lacking empathy, they either repress or shift their empathy. These individuals have personality abnormalities rather than being actual psychopaths. The reason is believed to be atypical behavior in the brain's pain and fear regions. Even so, these irregularities would bring uncontrolled faults into the programming of the ego without the balancing impact of spirit, which would then cause the ego to run wild and attract the attention of the legal and medical systems. Other spiritless persons who have healthy egos are better at hiding their lack of regret and empathy behind more sophisticated social training.

Conclusion

In this class of mankind, it is now clear why humans would be thought of as being robotic, shallow, predatory, and animalistic. We are not all the same on the inside; we are divided into divine beings and our polar opposites, made up of empty beings. People who deny the existence of spiritless people will continue to shake their heads in disbelief at actions they are forced to either ignore or understand. These individuals behave in accordance with their material predetermined nature, which is shaped by a variety of cues, sociality, and consciousness. They are spiritless in nature and can only accept things within their realm of understanding. Through my own experience, speaking with people, it's almost as if there is a consciousness barrier where certain information, words, or conversations do not click or comprehend into their brain. Once you say certain things about spiritual phenomena or some world affairs going on, they either go silent, switch conversations, leave, or have a few words to say and are uninterested in talking about the subject. But they will be quick to talk and converse about their favorite video game or movie for about 5 minutes. They lack open-minded thought and conversations and it seems like they always have a discomfort or weird feeling about what they are hearing. Sometimes they would freeze or feel bothered, basically like a glitch.

How Do You Know?

You are not spiritless if you have experienced even one spirit-specific quality. Such as empathy, love, wisdom, independent thinking, originality, uniqueness, inner search, love for nature, and etc. The very fact that you have wondered about it, that you are unsure of it, and that you want to know for certain demonstrates self-awareness and introspection—another quality of spirit. Whatever the case, it is preferable to accept that you do have spirit and focus on cultivating its qualities, such as intuition, empathy, and clarity, while also being conscious of your lower egocentric tendencies and not acting on them. The fact that you are reading this right now because you have a direct interest or desire to learn about the world at large, indicates you are a spirited being. If you are able to connect with and distinguish between the two polar opposites of this world, you are capable of understanding its limitations. It is best to consciously know where people's frequency resonates so you are able to adjust and grasp their reality. Going after everyone who is "spiritless" or spotting the individuals among them is not worthwhile since it simply makes you grow apprehensive. It is possible to see the diversity that all life possesses without losing sight of that unity. By fully appreciating each part of that unity we can live life in bliss and peace.

Angel Numbers

Angel numbers are numerical values that are used by divine power to send particular signals and guidance to people on Earth. The universe communicates with all of us. While we are here on Earth, the ascended masters and guardian angels watch over us and do their best to help us navigate through life, shape our reality, and alter our lives for the better. Angels help and communicate with us in a variety of ways, including synchronicities, our dreams, meditation, numbers, and through people. Angel numbers can provide us with both positive omens and warnings to keep in mind during negative times. You will continue to receive these divine and heavenly messages even after you have awakened; they will always be available to push us, assist us in growing, and direct us. In numerology, repeating sequences of numbers are referred to as "master numbers" and are a sign to pay attention to your mind, body, and soul. Examples of master numbers include 1111, 222, and 555. Observing the numbers is not an accident, regardless of whether you believe they are angels, the universe, or just your higher self calling to you. Angel numbers are also a sign of symptoms of awakening: you start to see how your life around you starts to manifest through your own thoughts, and the numbers help you keep your goals and dreams in check.

How Numerology Works

Each numerical value has a meaning, so when the numbers are put together they convey a message behind it. The position of a number, its relationship to other letters, and patterns determine its power. Similar to how we use numbers to rank certain stages and levels, these numbers are used for levels because of their mystical use of giving power to the world and things around us. Numbers convey messages in the same way letters create compounds of words, through their symbolic meaning relating to a power or source. By comprehending each single digit we can understand the spiritual and magical vibrations of the self. The dates of numerology go as far as 6th century CE and to the earliest of our antiquity. However, we have developed more into a less spiritual and aware aspect of ourselves that most do not pay attention to. The 6th-century BCE philosopher and mystic Pythagoras believed that numbers carried sacred codes and were divinely inspired and created. Behind each veil, there is a system of alchemical numerology that is employed to examine the innate rhythms of mathematics. Numbers may be used in a mystical sequence to transmit codes and divine messages from beyond, just like words can. Numbers also carry a vibration. The historical connections between astrology, astronomy, alchemy, and chemistry are equivalent in this regard. Mathematical formulas and numbers may be used to define the alchemy of time and consciousness.

In the modern world, divinatory practices like palmistry, tarot, and numerology are frequently linked to the occult. Early Gnostic occultism, early Christian mysticism, Pythagoras and his disciples (6th century B.C.), the Hebrew Kabbalah, the Indian Vedas, the Chinese "Circle of the Dead," and the Egyptian "Book of the Master of the Secret House" (Ritual of the Dead) are just a few examples of the ancient cultures and teachers whose elements are often discovered in modern numerology.

Historical Examples:
- The Kabbalah, a body of esoteric texts that explains Jewish mysticism, uses the 22 letters of the Hebrew alphabet to calculate a name's numerological value. After each letter and number are aligned, they are combined together. This method was initially employed by Kabbalistic philosophers to conceal the text of the Kabbalah from skeptics. Over time, it became a method for determining your career and place in life-based on your name.
- As stated by St. Augustine of Hippo (A.D. 354–430), "Numbers are the Universal language offered by the deity to humans as confirmation of the truth." He shared with Pythagoras that everything has a numerical connection and that it is either up to the mind to look for and explore these connections on its own, or the divine will show them to us.
- Pythagoras, a mathematician and philosopher from Ancient Greece, held that any number may be expressed as a single digit between one and nine. He believed that we could grasp the spiritual and magical vibrations of self by understanding the single numbers.
- The Chaldean method was used in Ancient Babylon and focused on how the numbers one through eight vibrated. In Chaldean, the number nine is holy and sacred. It symbolizes a connection to the divine and everything one could want in the world. The number 9 is recognised as the completion and ultimate number in numerology throughout the ancient world.

- The Indian numerology, sometimes referred to as Tamil numerology, has its roots in Tamil, a language native to Southern India. When calculating the results of this type of numerology, three crucial factors for each individual are taken into account. These three numbers are the name number, destiny number, and psychic number.

- Pythagoras himself was the one who discovered Western numerology, which is also known as Pythagorean numerology. In this version of numerology, each letter in the alphabet is given a specific number, which makes the calculation process simpler.

Numbers direct paths, coded messages, and even words, it is a means of communication using different variables. With the use of numerology, one may learn more about themselves, other individuals, and how they relate to the rest of the world.

Examples - Number 9

- The number "9" symbolizes "completion" since it is the last and highest value of a single-digit number. Considering it is the final of the single-digit numbers (also known as cardinal numbers in numerology) and possesses the highest value, the number nine is said to signify completion. That said, the number "9" represents a culmination of wisdom, experience, and vibrates with the energy of both ends and new beginnings. Since "9" is the highest single-digit number, you may infer the spiritual meaning of "new phase of awakening" and "end of a cycle" from the repeating sequence. It also carries the connotation of "higher self" owing to its value.

- **Using the number 9 as an example: (Biblical Perspective):** The number 9 is used 49 times in the Bible to represent the finality or completeness of God. Christ died at three in the afternoon, at the ninth hour of the day, to open the way to salvation to everyone. Only one of God's annual feast days, the Day of Atonement (Yom Kippur), requires believers to fast for one day. According to Leviticus 23:32, this special day, which many Jews consider to be the holiest day of the year, begins at sunset on day 9 of the seventh Hebrew month.

- According to Galatians 5:22–23, the number 9 also stands for the fruits of the Holy Spirit, which are faithfulness, gentleness, goodness, joy, kindness, patience, love, peace, and self-control. From a biblical point of view, the number on the calendar that corresponds to a significant day represents that particular event's number (in history).

Gematria:

- Gematria, which is very good at predicting certain events, is another example of using numerical values.

- Gematria (/ge'mertrie/); Hebrew: The practice of using an alphanumeric cipher to assign a numerical value to a name, word, or phrase is known as nuna or gimatria nona (plural nimuna or nixon'a, gimatriot). Depending on the cipher used, a single word can produce multiple values.

- In gematria, each numerical number has significance and meaning. It is calculated by combining words and letters to represent a particular number associated with its meaning.

- Gematria sums can be just a few words or a long series of calculations. The word 'n chai is a well-known short example of gematria cipher-based Hebrew numerology. This is made up of two letters that add up to 18, using the assignments in the Mispar gadol table. Because of this, the Jewish people consider the number 18 to be "lucky." Jewish people at certain events like weddings, would give sums of money that are multiples of 18 in order to wish a friend good luck.

Deity Examples - 9

- **Odin In Norse mythology:** Odin is also associated with the number nine because that is the number of days he spent hanging from the worldly tree 'Yggdrasil' before learning the runes.

- **Yggdrasil's "9" realms - The Tree of Life:** The number nine is also significant because, according to Norse cosmology, there are nine worlds that Yggdrasil supports. The Anglo-Saxon paganism charm known as the nine-herbs charm, as its name suggests, invokes nine herbs and also makes a rare reference to Woden.

- **Cultural Example "9":** In Chinese culture, the number nine (tt pinyin jiù) is regarded as a good number because it sounds like the word "long-lasting" (I pinyin jiü). Nine has a strong connection to the Chinese dragon, which is a symbol of power and magic. The dragon is described in terms of nine attributes, has nine forms, and has nine offsprings. It contains 117 scales, of which 36 are yin (feminine, earthly), and 81 are yang (masculine, Heavenly). All three integers have the same digital root of 9, and they are all multiples of 9 (9 13 = 117, 9 9 = 81, and 9 4 = 36)

Angel Numbers And Their Actual Meanings 1-9

1. **111 meaning:** In your journey, it is a sign of enlightenment and a message to follow your desires because angelic guidance is behind you. The number one signifies determination and independence, as well as the time of new beginnings.

2. **222 meaning:** The best is yet to come. Keep in mind that you are headed in the right direction. Your future manifestations and visualizations are yet to arrive. Two represents balance and the second stage is towards discovering your path.

3. **333 meaning:** Encouragement for your work and for making the right decisions in life. In the end, it is a symbol of confidence. The ascended masters who are with you and helping you also have a strong connection to the number 333. Three is the number of assurance and direction on your path.

4. **444 meaning:** It denotes the conclusion of one phase and the beginning of another. It can refer to a personal or spiritual transformation. The number four represents stability and discipline.

5. **555 meaning:** Period of transition when significant change is imminent. Spiritual guides whose mission is to support and rebuild you. It also symbolizes exploration and adventure. Five is the number of new opportunities and changes in one's life.

6. **666 meaning:** You are out of balance and order. Meaning to gather yourself and refocus, put your life in order. The number of the material's focus is six.

7. **777 meaning:** The time to reap the benefits of your efforts is indicated by this sign of divine guidance and order. You are making significant positive changes in your life, and you are on the right path to obtaining luck and abundance. 777 is regarded as the most divine number in numerology. Seven is a balance of peace and neutrality.

8. **888 meaning:** Success, money, and good fortune is coming. You are heading in the right direction, according to the universe. Eight is addressed with infinity and boundless love and energy in the universe.

9. **999 meaning:** New awakening phase and the conclusion of a cycle. Related to maturity, and demonstrates your higher self is yet to make a move. The number of completed tasks and new paths entered is nine.

Angel Numbers And Their Meanings: 10-22

1. **1010 meaning:** A new beginning signifying the arrival of something new. It indicates that you are on the right path and experiencing a spiritual awakening. When you see the number 1010, you are experiencing a spiritual awakening. The angel number 1010 is a representation of self-realization. It indicates that you are on the right track and will soon discover who you really are.

2. **1111 meaning:** Indicates that you are going through a major awakening and that angelic energies are being backed by powers that you are not able to see. When you see the number 1111, you may sigh with relief and power, because it confirms that everything in your universe right now is on schedule and being directed by the divine.

3. **1212 meaning:** Discovery and awakening. Encountering the number 1212 indicates that your guardian angels are watching over, defending, and helping you. The angel number 1212 may indicate that you are soon to experience prosperity in your life.

4. **1313 meaning:** Good is yet to come. Represents possibilities to learn from the past and fresh beginnings, 1313 is a symbol of fresh starts. The universe is presenting you with a fresh start so that you can correct your previous errors.

5. **1414 meaning:** It's time to take action! Concentrate on your needs and goals. Your guardian angels are reminding you with the angel number 1414 that you will need to lay a strong foundation for your future endeavors.

6. **1515 meaning:** Assurance from the angels of protection. It is said that seeing the number 1515 represents a spiritual message from your guardian angel. According to Psalm 91:11, God sends angels to Earth to guide us and deliver messages. Your guardian angels are assuring you that they are looking over and guarding you with the angel number 1515.

7. **1616 meaning:** Fulfill your potential. Concentrate on the good aspects of life and your family.

8. **1717 meaning:** Reassurance of soul contract agreement and soul purpose. A sign that you are heading in the right direction to accomplishing your goals.

9. **1818 meaning:** The universe is entirely committed to helping you achieve your goals. Something is keeping an eye on you. If you are given the angel number 1818, the universe will fully back your goals.

10. **1919 meaning:** You are connected divinely to the highest (ascended masters). If you see the number 1919, it means that you have a connection to the holy. You will be able to achieve your highest goals through this connection.

11. **2020 meaning:** Prepare yourself for what lies ahead. Your guardian angels are instructing you to mentally and physically prepare for the upcoming changes in your life.

12. **2121 meaning:** Have faith in yourself. It tells you that your thoughts are like seeds about to grow and that things will go in the way you want them to. The angel number 2121 represents authority and prosperity. It motivates you to believe in your abilities and self-worth.

13. **2222 meaning:** Good things are still to come, as destiny is determined by these numbers. Follow a specific course of action. The number 2222 from the angels is a good sign for you. It's a sign that a time of peace and stability is about to begin.

14. **144 meaning:** Reminder you are among the anointed ones. Stick to your purpose and enlighten the world.

As they direct you in the right direction, pay attention to any additional meanings or indications of warnings provided by angel numbers or other numerical sequences. These sets of angel numbers can also be unique to different people. To express these signals, the following numbers were all calculated and created by combinations of their numerical values. Everyone also has their own signature number—an angel number—with which they are most in tune with and to which they sense a strong connection. Your life path is essentially represented by these numbers.

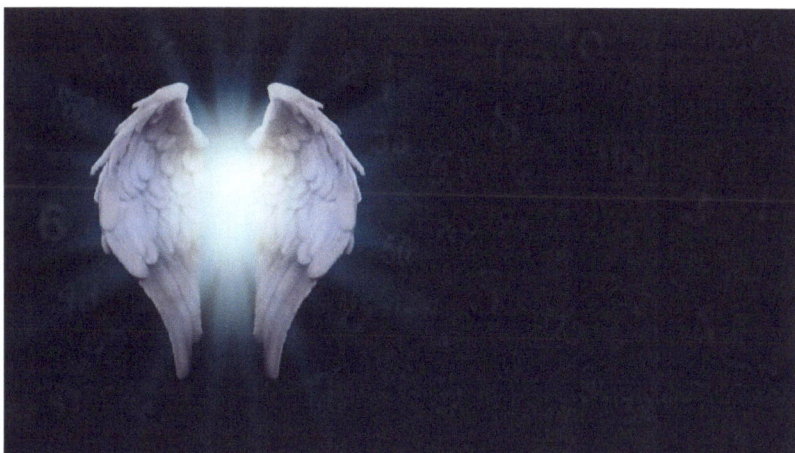

Solfeggio Frequencies And Their Functions

Solfeggio frequencies are electromagnetic tones that are utilized for consciousness expansion and healing. By focusing on specific tones that can heal and energize our electromagnetic field, these frequencies are able to rejuvenate and raise the vibration in our bodies. Like batteries, our bodies can recharge themselves with supplied energy and frequencies. Solfeggio frequencies serve as the foundation for several historical religious music traditions that date all the way back to the eighth century, such as the Gregorian and Indian Sanskrit chants. Everything in our universe is moving and vibrating, including our bodies, atoms, inanimate objects, molecules, thoughts, and sounds. We must align ourselves with the frequency of the planet itself, which has its own (6-30 Hz). Solfeggio frequencies are among the specific sound patterns that interact with your brain to cause bodily vibrations. The vibrations can have benefits on your mental, emotional, and physical health. These frequencies adjust you to the rhythms and tones that structure the premise of the Universe.

Albert Einstein once said, **"Everything in our Universe is vibration."**

The human ear has a certain range of vibrations that it can pick up in a second. In sound science, the term "frequency" refers to the number of vibrations per second, which is measured in Hz. Solfeggio frequencies are based on the notion of specific sounds', which span from 174 Hz to 963 Hz. The fact that our thoughts have a big influence on both our mental and physical health is now largely accepted. Ultrasonic sound is used by some medical devices to help heal bone regeneration and speed up the healing of fractured bones. Similar tools are also used to tighten and tone the skin and remove tummy fat. Having said that, research has shown that exposure to certain frequencies can rewire your brain and increase your ability to manage emotions. Listening to harmony sounds (such as meditation music) at such frequencies is very beneficial since they enhance healing, unlock DMT, enable downloads, and unlock DNA.

Solfeggio frequencies

Fork Names	Frequency (in Hz)	Chakra	Characteristics
UT	369	Root	Liberate from guilt and fear
RE	417	Sacral	Undoing Situations and Facilitate Change
MI	528	Naval	Transformations and Miracles (DNA Repair)
FA	639	Heart	Connecting/Relationships
SOL	741	Throat	Expression
LA	852	Brow	Awakening Intuition
	963	Crown	Connect with light and spirit

Negatives of Certain Frequencies

The elites of Hollywood and around the world are using music and sounds to influence behavior by targeting the brain with frequencies that contain harmful and symbolic lyrics. According to studies, the impacts of particular frequencies can alter the body's rhythm and lead to irregular heartbeats. A person can get up and do something, such as act impulsively or commit a crime, in reaction to these frequencies. It negatively stimulates the brain and completely impairs cognitive function. People who listen to music are heavily influenced by what it contains, such as the symbols, lyrics, and also the frequencies.

The frequency played in a great deal of mainstream music, A440 hertz, has been demonstrated to be harmful since it can alter emotions like rage and excitement and increase dopamine levels in the brain. Due to the dopamine surge, it changes the brain's basic functioning system and becomes addictive. It asks the brain for more and more of the same satisfaction, almost like a drug. Like a spell, mainstream music's use of negative and impulsive frequencies is a weapon that makes users addicted and alters their thoughts and actions in response to them. People can be seen running and jumping around in a club or party because the frequencies being generated alter the body's rhythm and increase heart rate. We are programmed to listen to frequencies that are harmful rather than those that are beneficial. The problem is that everyone has spent their whole lives listening to static, which increases the likelihood of harm. However, positive tonal frequencies like 174 Hz, 285 Hz, 396 Hz, 417 Hz, 528 Hz, 639 Hz, 741 Hz, and others can be used to treat it. Natural sound melodies coming directly from musical instruments are much more put into harmony than artificialized frequencies generated from bass. Natural music allows positive frequencies to flow through rather than ones that alter the consciousness. Singing, listening, or creating nature music, has positive biological and psychological effects. By providing a healthy distraction and requiring us to be more mindful, it can help us relax.

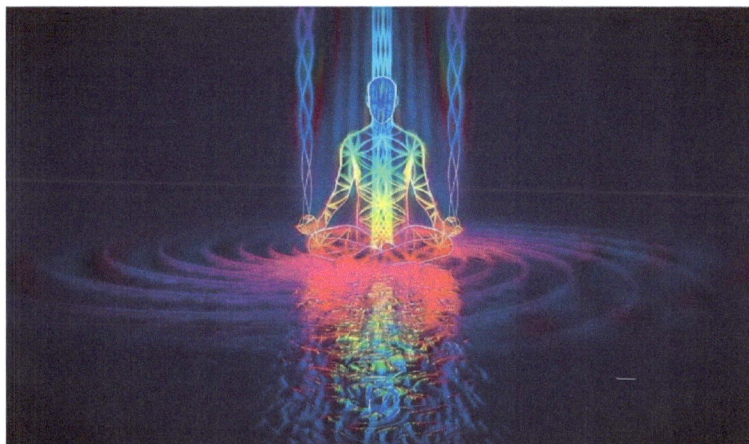

Types of Frequency Hz And Their Functions

1. **40 Hz**: Gamma brain waves and memory stimulation have been linked to sound at 40 hertz. Helps improve focus and memory. CROWN CHAKRA

2. **174 Hz**: One of the Solfeggio frequencies is 174 hertz. This tone is used in alternative medicine and in sacred music. 174 hertz aids in stress and pain reduction. ROOT CHAKRA

3. **285 Hz:** Solfeggio frequency, 285 hertz, is thought to aid in the healing of cuts, burns, and other physical wounds. The body is encouraged to heal itself in the event of an injury when 285 hertz sound frequencies are used. ROOT CHAKRA

4. **396Hz:** Sound frequency is linked to removing anxiety and other negative emotions. ROOT/HEART/SACRAL CHAKRA

5. **417 Hz:** Focuses on getting rid of negative energy, like the energy of past trauma or the negative energy in the surrounding environment. The goal of 417-hertz therapy is to open the sacral chakra and break down emotional blocks. ROOT/HEART/SACRAL CHAKRA

6. **528 Hz:** One of the most well-known and popular Solfeggio frequencies is 528 hertz, which is a love frequency. Native Americans have utilized this musical tone, which is also referred to as the "miracle note." Also used for past life regression meditation. HEART/CROWN CHAKRA

7. **639 Hz:** The heart chakra is used by the sound frequency 639 hertz. The purpose of this sound frequency is to increase achievement and positive feelings. HEART CHAKRA

8. **852 Hz:** 852 hertz sound therapy is a tone that is associated with redirecting the mind. Such as overthinking, intrusive thoughts, and negative thought patterns. CROWN CHAKRA

9. **963 Hz:** Sound frequencies of 963 hertz are linked to spiritual growth and pineal gland activation. The frequency of 963 hertz, also referred to as the "pure miracle tone" and the "frequency of the gods," facilitates the activation of the crown chakra and a connection to the universal source. THIRD EYE/CROWN CHAKRA

Small Tips for Self-Improvement

This list is for you! Cultivate these habits and tips that can help you improve your life, increase your vibration, and things to explore and look into.

1. **Loving yourself /Self Appreciation:** Cultivate having a high regard for your own well-being and happiness.
2. **Getting Sunlight (Sun-gazing):** Helps improve consciousness and health and boost the body's vitamin supply.
3. **Grounding (Barefoot):** Increases vibration being directly close to Earth, heals the body, and helps balance and core chakras.
4. **Nofap (Semen Retention):** Helps develop sexual discipline, creates sacredness, increases focus, increases energy, and helps battle sex or porn addictions.
5. **Mirror Talk (Reflection):** Helps reflect, manifest, and affirm things you want to come into your life. Builds self-awareness and rationality in decision-making.
6. **Affirmations (Positivity, Dreams, Good Karma):** Minimizes negative thinking and shows life in a positive perspective.
7. **Shadow Work:** Working with your unconscious mind to uncover and heal the parts of yourself that you repress and hide from yourself.
8. **Cleansing:** Includes detoxing, saging, and isolating from negative energy. Cleansing overall helps remove negative toxins or energy and bring in positive ones.
9. **Connecting With Animals and Nature:** Connects to the crown chakra, raises vibration, and connects you closer to the universe and your own spirituality. Teaches you to appreciate and love life the way it is in its natural state.
10. **Working Out:** Keeps you active, healthy and in shape. A healthy body = a healthy mind. (gym, pushups, running, stretching, burpees, jump-rope, sports, etc.)
11. **Investing Money:** Investing is an effective way to put your money to work and potentially build wealth. (business, health, crypto, stocks, savings, emergency funds, etc.)
12. **Ending Bad Habits:** Identify your own triggers and things that slow you down from your poor behaviors or habits. Practice mindfulness. (for e g, gossiping, procrastinating, etc.)

13. **Planning Your Days:** Find something to do every day that will help you be productive. Maintain self-discipline by doing something meaningful every day and inspire yourself to reach higher goals.

14. **Cold Showers:** Boosts immunity, increases metabolism, increases blood circulation, combats sexual urges, combats depression, relieves localized pain, allows less access of fluoride into pores, and is overall healthier. (even if it's just the last 20 seconds of your regular shower)

15. **Not relying on Relationships/Companionships for Happiness:** Love yourself never seek validation or expectations for others to love you. Be yourself, love yourself, and have confidence in your own body.

16. **Not comparing yourself to others:** Compare yourself to yesterday and become a better person. You are the reflection of others and others you judge. People are continually reflecting your consciousness back to you, allowing you to evolve and change your perceptions of both yourself and other people.

17. **Helping Others:** Cultivate empathy, raise the heart chakra, be a good role model, and increase good karma to attract the same back.

18. **Not Trying to Impress People:** Impress yourself from yesterday and become the best YOU. If we seek approval from others on a regular basis, we may begin to assume that our worth is dependent upon what other people think of us.

19. **Breathing In From Your Nose:** Breathing through your nose improves circulation, humidifies your nasal passages, and acts as a natural filter for toxins.

20. **Cleaning Your Room/House:** Healthy discipline cultivates good habits and positive attraction. Discipline comes from the Solar Plexus chakra and manages yourself for the better.

21. **Taking Breaks of Social Media (or quit it):** Reduce the amount of useless time you spend on social media and do things more productive. Anxiety and depression can be significantly reduced by taking a week off from social media, overall improving your quality of life.

22. **Making up your bed:** Making your bed is a disciplined practice that raises our solar plexus chakra and improves sleep quality.

23. **Eating Healthier and Learning to Cook:** People who eat well live longer and are less likely to have serious health issues like obesity, type 2 diabetes, and heart disease. Making your own food helps you develop fundamental life skills, cut back on processed food, and consciously choose healthy foods for your body. Try being vegan if you are on a spiritual journey, it helps with consuming higher vibrational foods, cultivates ethical conduct, empathy, and also creates a light body for more spiritual experiences.

24. **Weekly Walks:** Increases clarity, balances chakras, increases vibration, connects to nature, increases activity, increases mindfulness and improves health. (in nature, use no headphones/AirPods)

25. **Learning How to Defend Yourself:** The weak are taken advantage of by those in positions of influence or power in our harsh reality. Keep your ground and stick up for what you believe in. Your confidence and self-esteem rise when you are able to defend yourself. (verbally and physically)

26. **Drinking Water Daily:** Getting enough water every day is important for your health. Increases energy, relieves fatigue, increases mental clarity, promotes weight loss, keeps you alkaline, flushes out toxins, and improves skin. (drink 2-4 liters a day, avoid fluoride, drink natural spring)

27. **Wisdom:** Reading, learning, and seeking more knowledge.

28. **Finding and Fulfilling Purpose:** Working or seeking a higher purpose or end goal.

29. **Awareness:** Going within, finding more about yourself and around your environment.

30. **Self-Destructing Habits:** Quitting/moderating drugs/alcohol - all low vibrational which hinders cognitive function and overall health.

31. **Healthy Choices:** Quitting/moderating caffeine and sugary drinks - supplanting negativity with healthier options.

32. **Meditating:** Meditation increases mindfulness, consciousness, clarity, mood, stress, creativity, etc.

33. **Giving To The Less Fortunate:** Helping others in need always creates good karma and something good for others to remember. It creates a sense of belonging, value, and makes others appreciative.

34. **Cutting Out Bad Friends and Family:** You are who you hang around with, protect your energy and surround yourself with high vibrational beings who are productive, helpful,

and respect you. Cut off all toxic people out of your life, you will open yourself up to forgiveness and learn from your past. You will also see a better quality of life and won't have people pull you down into negativity.

35. **Minimalism:** Avoiding the unnecessary; simplicity is more important than complications that will cause stress.

36. **Goals:** Having a plan for things you wanna do and work towards it. Always have something you want to achieve even after an accomplished objective.

37. **Learning:** Find something you're good at and excel. (e.g., remote, skill coding, music, designing, marketing, etc.)

38. **Protect Your Energy:** Be aware of what you're doing with your valuable time and energy, as well as who you're around.

39. **Know Your Roles:** Acting in a manner that is appropriate for your gender. (man or woman)

40. **Respect and Admiration:** Respect fosters positive relationships and creates a positive environment. Also always show respect to nature and wildlife; it is our economy, society, and underpins our existence.

Spiritual Meanings

Here is a collection of spiritual interpretations that connect to the paranormal signals found in our physical world. Everything is spiritual, also, everything that occurs above also occurs below. We are given signs and messages from the divine every single day of our lives. We receive unlimited daily downloads emanating from the divine consciousness of our universe; however, we must be in tune and one with the universe in order to comprehend these messages. Everything has a spiritual significance, and our individual downloads show us how to apply these messages to our awareness and inner self. Over the course of years, these downloads from the divine are based on my own writings and thoughts. This will help in developing a spiritual worldview on events and an understanding of the spiritual world.

1. **Say "I love you water" affirmation, to your water:** Setting a good motive can boost your spiritual currency and well-being. The crystalline structure of water stores memories and can interact with you to raise your vibration. This affirmation is potent because water exchanges messages and emotions with water-based cells in your body. Dr. Masaru Emoto's work indicates that when water is exposed to positive words and intentions, beautiful symmetrical crystal forms grow when the water is frozen, however when water is subjected to negative words and intentions, disorderly, asymmetrical structures form.

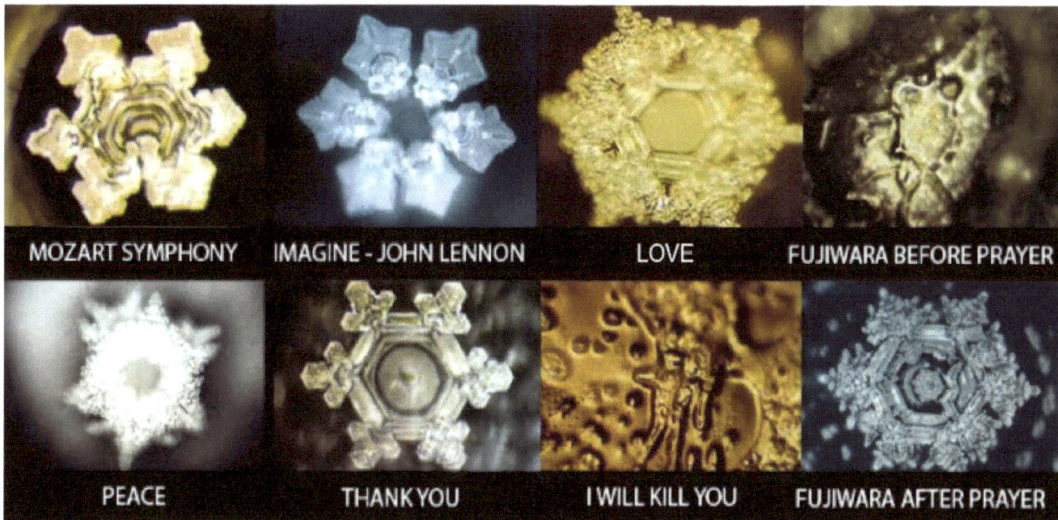

2. **Spiritual Effect of Sleeping With Window Open:** You invite unwanted spirits into your home when you go to sleep with the door or window open. Throughout Europe, this belief was prevalent.

3. **Spiritual Effect of Sleeping Beside Mirrors:**
   - The mirror close to your bed might be an entryway for spirits, a doorway that they can use to enter and exit. The historical backdrop of mirrors goes back hundreds of years.
   - In astral projection, a mirror in your house is an entrance, where you can communicate with various assortments of spirits. Mirrors can restore a sense of DeJaVu by acting as portals.
   - The soul and physical appearance are both reflected in mirrors.

4. **Spiritual Meaning Behind Birthmarks:** Birthmarks can represent a story from your past life—a death or a wound, depending on the shape—or both. In previous incarnations, it may also represent a specific tribe or group. Birthmarks can be connected to animal spirits as well as astrological representations of the cosmos.

5. **Spiritual Meaning Behind People Deflecting Eye Contact:** If others avoid looking at you or stumble when speaking to you a lot, it means that your light and force have an effect on their soul and auric/energy. This indicates that the light in your aura, eyes, and body affects the other person. The energy of others can be feared by the light force of chosen ones, which brings a message into the subconscious mind on a spiritual level.

6. **Spiritual Meaning Behind Karma:** All of your bad behavior from the past will come back to you once you awaken. A spiritual or awakened person experiences karma three times more strongly since they are aware of its effects and recognise their acts have consequences on deeper levels. This is why high vibration is essential for attracting good karma.

7. **Spiritual Meaning Behind Ear Ringing:** The sensation that your ears are ringing is brought on by the calls of your ancestors and the universe's resonance with your energy. These pitches have vibrational frequencies that link you together. Additionally, it is a sign of a spiritual awakening. Ear ringing is also an angelic message and call to communicate with you. This refers to a psychic symptom.

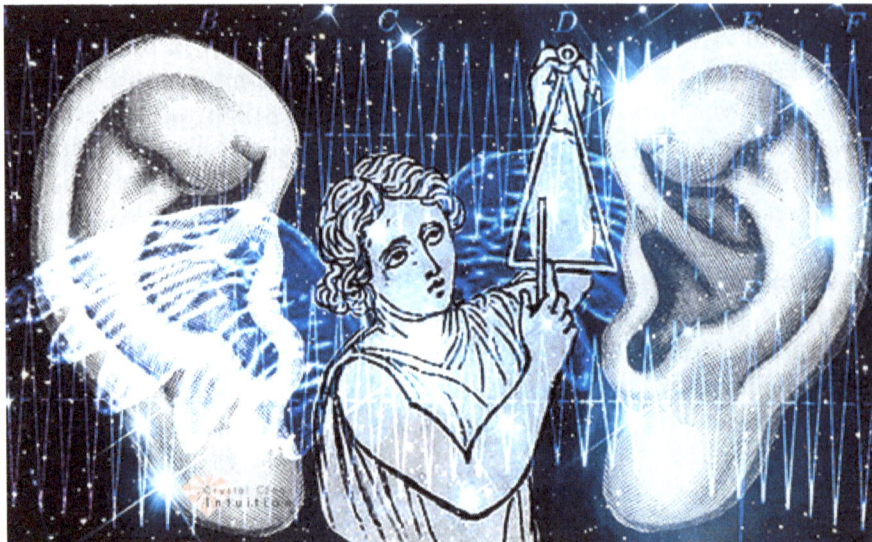

8. **Spiritual Meaning Behind Seeing Sparks:** A sign that your third eye has opened to the spiritual world is seeing sparks. Sparks represent the fine veil between the physical world and the spiritual. It indicates that the psychic abilities are lining up and is an indication of spiritual awakening.

9. **Spiritual Meaning Behind Name Calling in Dreams:** If someone calls your name in your dreams, it means that a messenger is trying to get in touch with you. It indicates that something wants your attention. Pay attention to this because it will reveal clues about who you are, and it could also be deities attempting to connect with you in the spiritual realm.

10. **Spiritual Meaning Behind Sharingan:** The Sharingan is a spiritual concept that can be brought to life through a variety of spiritual third-eye enhancement techniques. These techniques focus on developing reflexes, energy reading, perceptive abilities, and the ability to identify deities and auras. This ability has been recognised by people who are gifted at reading energy.

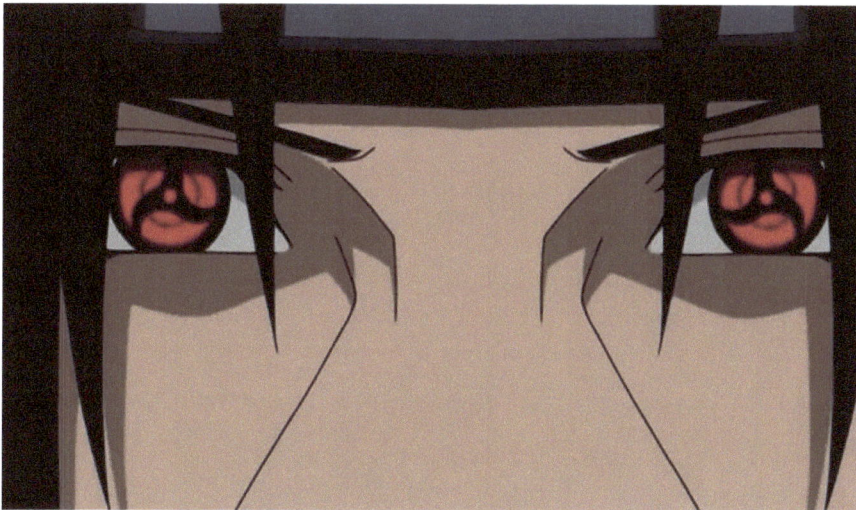

11. **Spiritual Meaning Behind Buzzing Cicadas:** Resurrection and spiritual recognition are represented by cicadas. The transcendental vocals of cicadas are designed to resonate with your own vibration. According to ancient beliefs, Plato asserts that cicadas can also act as a wake-up call or a call to communicate with the dead spirits. Cicadas also represent change, rebirth, renewal, and transformation.

12. **Spiritual Meaning Behind Astral Projection or Dream Scars:** In order to avoid scars and potential paranormal activity, astral projection should only be carried out in a high vibration, well-fasted, and clear environment. This is because a battle in the spiritual realm can remotely transcend into physical life. Although spirits are all-knowing, they can only consume you if you allow them to and enter a passage for them to contact.

13. **Spiritual Meaning Behind Sexual Dreams:** Applied to both men and women. Demonic sexual demons are vying for power when a person has lustful energy in their dreams. These spirits, also known as succubus and incubus, have the ability to seduce people sexually in their dreams while draining their energy. Having an excessive amount of lust and sexual pleasure saps your mental and physical energy and makes it harder to think rationally.

14. **Spiritual Meaning Behind The Medusa Effect:** Throughout many conversations, there are a lot of people who pause, stop, or gaze. During the discourse, the person is unable to withstand the grip of the light; this is an indication of a warring spirit within them. It is a spiritual entanglement that causes the subconscious mind to freeze. This usually happens to light workers who regularly interact with low vibrational people; the resentful spirits inside the person are aware of the light and truth you carry.

15. **Spiritual Meaning Behind - Targeted Advertising:** Have you ever wondered the reason why your phone knows exactly what you're thinking and displays relevant advertisements or messages without you saying a word or searching for anything? There are two things to consider: First, the government keeps an eye on everything you do. Second, there is a spiritual significance to synchronicities that always occur in reality regarding your own thoughts.

- Google mimics the conversations you're likely to have. This is due to the fact that they have a "digital voodoo doll" of each individual to conduct an analysis of you, your routines, and other factors. Targeted ads are not a coincidence; smartphones can read your thoughts. Google and Facebook are able to create what ex-Googler ethicist Harris calls a "little voodoo doll, avatar-like version" of people in order to predict which advertisements they will click on and which products they will buy since they have gathered so much information about you and your habits.

- Through spiritual synchronicities, our phones constantly display messages and signs that correspond to our own thoughts. These are spirits collaborating with the algorithm to project your thoughts onto your phone/device. Because our phones and technology are so ingrained in us, it's almost simple for spirits or even angels to communicate electronically without having to be physically present with us.

16. **Spiritual/Truth Meaning Behind Reincarnation:** Reincarnation is the process of failing to reach the Tree of Life or returning to this world for a purpose. Like a video game, your soul will keep coming back until you get it right. You don't have just one life; you've had many, but your memory has been whittled away. However, there are gifted individuals who are able to accurately recall specific details and facts from previous lives. Start accumulating good karma and working toward your divine purpose because your current existence also serves as a setup for your future life. Everyone has a soul purpose—what they came here to do—and not everyone succeeds. This idea, which is truly the Tree of Life, has been a part of many religions and cultures for thousands of years.

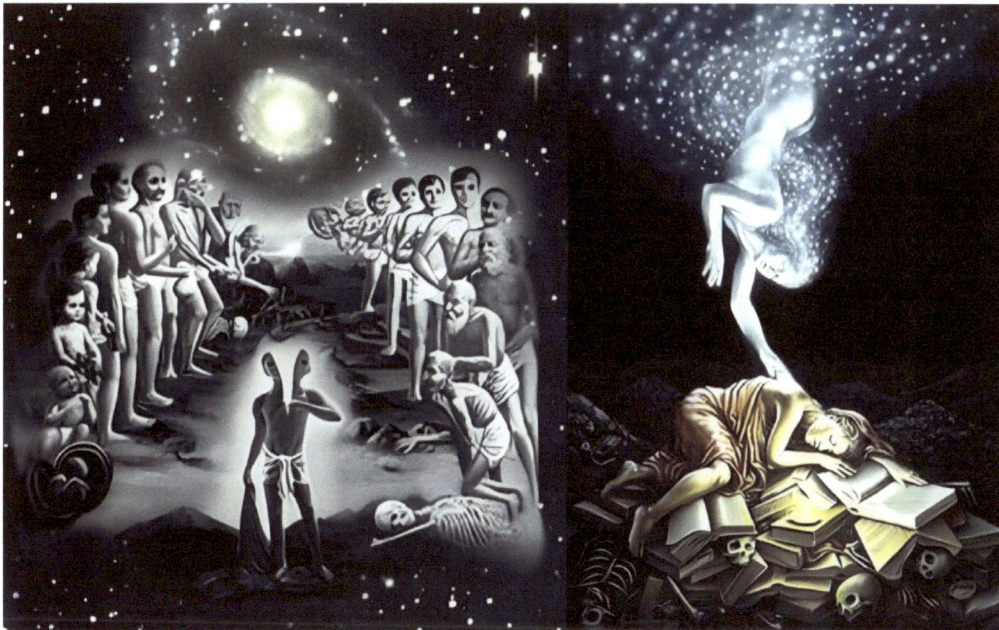

17. **Soul Stages:** How a person lives, thinks, acts, and rationalizes in this world is influenced by their soul age. A person must progress through a series of soul stages before achieving their ultimate goal of completeness.

Infant Souls

- The need for immediate survival is the primary focus of infant souls. They thrive in simple, natural settings like remote tribes, rural, or pastoral settings. The simplest needs are the primary focus of infant souls. They can either adapt to modern society or remain in an environment of primitive culture. Some people could be classified as psychopathic or as having developmental issues. This is due to the fact that an infant soul has not yet matured to experience or comprehend more advanced complexes of reality because they have yet to operate, resonate, and develop into a high consciousness.

- An infant soul has not yet learned the fundamental aspects of life and morality. Infant souls are impulsive, naive, and "pre-conventional," behaving impulsively or out of habit with little to no thought for the repercussions. They lack social awareness and self-control, making them capable of engaging in unethical or illicit behavior without feeling guilty about it. Due to their difficulty adapting to modern society, individuals could wind up in psychiatric or prison settings. They may be lacking in some principles, character qualities, or all-around competencies, but they are completely innocent and have no agenda.

Baby Souls

- Baby souls begin to grasp an understanding and think about the morals of right and wrong. Baby souls often follow orders and conform to the general masses as they focus on themselves with a great deal of safety, security, structure, and order. They generally follow and abide by the laws and live according to their environment. They like to live in communities that are highly principled and civilized and do not generate much independent thought or critical thinking.

- Considering their ideas and behavior are heavily governed by rules, they are generally highly traditionalist, orthodox, noble, moralistic, religiously devoted, and conscientious about law and order.

- They often give in to urges and temptations, sometimes throw tantrums, and sometimes break rules, but then they feel guilty and ashamed about it. They are able to develop their understanding of morals and the consequences of their actions to a limited extent. Although they have little insight into the reasons behind people's actions, they are acutely aware of the rights and wrongs of their own.

Young Souls

- Young souls place an emphasis on personal growth. Although they are still influenced by mainstream trends, they start to develop their own interests and begin to think for themselves. Young souls have a lot of energy, are outgoing, ambitious, competitive, and even some of them will be very interested in politics and the state of the world. Young souls do not operate with a spiritual conscience, they operate more within the ego than the other stages. They are generally attracted to worldly pleasures, fashion, power, glory and materialism. They can be stubborn and blind through materialistic views, as this soul stage is driven by the ego and allows the ego to self-adapt and be in more control.

- Many young souls aren't sure about their view or innate purpose in life, they just go with the flow, and may show little or no interest in things beyond this physical reality. They tend to fear death more than the other stages due to their state of uncertainty. Young souls tend to be extremely opinionated and exhibit little open-mindedness. They believe that their own point of view is the only one that is correct and ideal because they are more ego-driven. They are aware of their own agenda, behaviors, and justifications but never challenge them.

Mature Souls

- Mature souls are more calculated and reflective than young souls. They often question reality, grow self-awareness, operate more within empathy, and have a desire to be unique and authentic. Instead of chasing materialistic things, they operate a balance in cultivating spiritual things since they begin a reasoning to explore more to this universe. Mature consciousness is self-aware of the ego, egotistical tendencies, and no longer operates within the ego. They are able to accommodate multiple perspectives and different ambitions and reject narrow-minded views. They begin to understand different people's perspectives for their reasonings and have fixed opinions.

- Mature souls search for deeper meaning and self-knowledge, whether through art, psychology, philosophy, or spirituality. This is sparked by this loss of solid ground, which can be extremely stressful. Mature souls are prone to doing a lot of soul-searching and tend to question everything, even their own motives. They start to look past the physical reality, tend to get frustrated with people's motives and lack of empathy, and want to get down to the truth about the world.

Old/Ancient Soul

- Ancient souls tend to have a complete drive for wisdom, innovations, and knowledge. They are people ahead of their time and have more of an expression of inner peace and freedom. Sometimes old souls may feel alienated due to their interests in advanced subjects, rather than being interested in materialism or entertainment. They have moved beyond the stresses of mature souls and only want to be maintained within peace.

- They are more steady, measured, calm, and peaceful than younger souls are, unattached to cultural norms and societal institutions, confident in their own existence, inner resources, and have compassion for others. On the other hand, it may be quite depressing to discover oneself in a society that is so conflicting, chaotic, and shallow. Old souls are typically the philosophers of our age, teachers or masters, leading the new wave for the next generation.

- For old souls, full self-expression and satisfaction are the goals of life. In their later stages, old souls become conscious participants in the growth of all that is, and they often emphasize the need to share spiritual knowledge while showing great compassion.

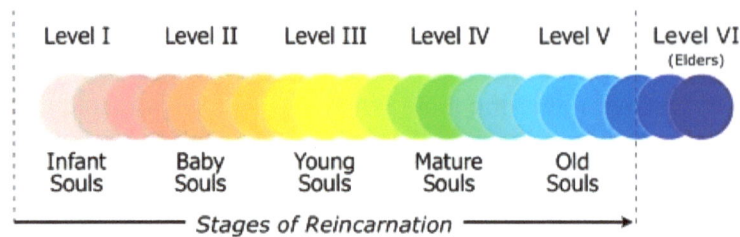

#	LEVEL	COLOR
1	Level I: Beginner	White
2	Level 1: Beginner	Off-white Gray / Grayish with tints of Pink
3	Level II: Lower Intermediate	White and Reddish Pink
4	Level II: Lower Intermediate	Light Orange Yellow with tints of White
5	Level III: Intermediate	Yellow
6	Level III & IV	Deep Gold / Gold with tints of Green
7	Level IV: Upper Intermediate	Green or Brownish Green
8	Level V: Advanced	Light Blue; Light Blue with Gold; Green or Brown tints
9	Level V & VI	Deep Blue
10	Level VI: Highly Advanced	Deep Blue with tints of Purple
11	Higher Levels	Purple

18. Letter People

- People with ADD, ADHD, and Asperger's syndrome are referred to as "The Letter People." These conditions are not caused by damaged genes, but rather by a limited reprogramming of a third-dimensional reality and the development of new multidimensional skills. It is a combination of improved bodies with improved genes and souls incarnating in these bodies from various parts of the universe. The DNA activation is influenced by the different frequencies and vibrations that the souls possess based on their evolutionary status. Letter people have difficulty communicating between the two halves of their brains and use one side of their brain to solve the same problem. Others claim to be dysfunctional, but it could be a way to free up brain space for more difficult higher-level and non-traditional learning tasks.

- Letter people are said to have different bodies and nervous systems, like an upgraded nerve system, the ability to see more colors between shades, acute taste and hearing senses, and frequency sensitivity. Additionally, the brains of "letter people" contain higher levels of acetylcholine and dopamine.

- The children having contact described by Homo Noeticus: They have telepathic abilities, which include superior mental abilities, a direct connection to higher awareness, enhanced DNA, photographic memories, extreme sensitivity to light and emotion, faster neuron responses, and high-quality nonverbal communication.

19. Extraterrestrial DNA and Advanced Intelligence Among Us - Looks at Data

- The biological identity of the human DNA programmer remains a mystery. "Then God said, and now we will make human beings, they will be like us and resemble us," the Christian Bible says in Genesis. DNA programming and extraterrestrial modification are suggested by this genesis clue.

- An "advanced civilization transported the seeds of life in a spaceship" is described by Francis Crick, co-founder of the DNA molecule and author of "Life Itself." These genes are unique to no other species on the planet. The enigma of biology: All 223 genes with sideways insertions of genetic material are linked to better mental health.

- According to geneticists, certain DNA dating methods can reveal the number of recently added genes to the human genome. According to Lloyd Pye's Intervention Theory, this kind of information has been hidden. Individual encounters from a 13-year-old named Canada, explains how extraterrestrial beings were interested in us humans and needed something with genetic qualities. The fact that few other children have the same experiences is a very strange sign.

- Human DNA raises the question of whether it is controlled by an extraterrestrial code that reveals our true origins. Maxim A. Makukov and Vladimir Shcherbak, two scientists, assert that our genetic code was altered by intelligent signals that were sent to the human race millions of years ago from outside the solar system. Compared to a brief extraterrestrial radio transmission, a biological seti would have a greater chance and longevity of detecting extraterrestrial life. Additionally, there are recognisable hallmarks of artificiality in our DNA. Maxim A. Makukov and Vladimir Shcherbak argue that patterns are basically resistant to any form of natural origin.

- According to Hawaiian University doctor William Brown, historical evidence of genetic manipulation suggests that extraterrestrial intervention occurred. The fusion of DNA molecules does not occur naturally. Human DNA contains numerous indications of genetic manipulation, indicating that advanced technology was used to alter the genomes.

- According to Dr. Roger Leir, alien or extraterrestrial interventions in our minds and bodies are to blame for the rapid advancement of the human species. This explains the generation's advancements and widespread awakening. In no less than 40 years of formative stages in children, it has expanded vigorously to 60-80% with talking, walking, and so on. The terrestrial consciousness of newborns is more awakened.

- Medical research at the University of California is one example of these changes of evidence. Some young children had 24 switches on active codons, whereas there are typically 20 in young children. With 24 active codons, these children were disease-free and had a stronger immune system.

- The more intelligent children in China, such as Nong Yousui, and other known advanced beings worldwide are an illustration of this. According to scientists, multiple mutations must occur simultaneously.

20. ADHD and Indigo Children

- Indigo children are children who are thought to have unique, out-of-the-ordinary, and occasionally supernatural abilities or traits. These beliefs are interpreted in a variety of ways, from the idea that they are the next stage in human evolution and have paranormal abilities like telepathy, to the belief that they are more creative and empathetic than their peers.

- Dr. William Brown explains the changes, pointing out that genetic modification is currently taking place and is in fact creating new humans. Children with autism, ADD, and Indigo Children, have an exponential increase in this. They are able to perceive the world in multiple dimensions thanks to the new genetic architecture. Research indicates that dormant genetic regions are being incorporated into the biological system, causing us all to become more aware. The DNA molecule's atomic structure contains the information. It can be accessed more quickly and produces traits similar to savants. The DNA modification is more of a genome re-modeling to make dormant areas accessible again.

21. Extraterrestrial (ET) Phenomenon

- Around the world, people of various ages, beliefs, races, and cultures communicate with extraterrestrials from past lives. Examples include a wide variety of non-human forms like Felines, Grays, Sirians, Mantids, and others. The interpretation of ET species requires careful consideration because there are multiple species and distinct perceptions of them that should be categorized. It's possible that there are more than 165 species of Grays and several distinct hybrids, each of which requires a unique understanding. Trust your own experiences because people's experiences may differ because of their own connections and understandings.

- This planet has been visited by extraterrestrials for thousands of years. The results of terrestrial species and prehistoric beings, such as giant fossils and alien scriptures, are confirmed by archaeological studies.

- The serpent extraterrestrial god in mythology can be traced back thousands of years. Such as the feathered serpent deity of ancient Mesoamerican culture known as Quetzalcoatl. The Sumerian serpent deities known as the Ningishzida and Bamu are another source.

- The hints and evidence are present throughout all of history, mythology, archaeology, anthropology, and the Bible. Personal encounters with extraterrestrials by adults and children are crucial in distinguishing life beyond Earth.

- This topic is enlightened by well-documented cases and personal experiences from indigenous cultures. The Ruwa UFO incident in 1994 is one example. In indigenous cultures, such as the Aborigines, who regard the "Mantid" or "Mantis" as gods and refer to them as "Mamoo," is referred to as an extraterrestrial being that is recognised by many people all over the world.

- Children who have an 'enhanced pineal gland' have drawings and detailed experiences of extraterrestrials, making them more connected to the spiritual realm. Native cultures and the Indian god Krishna are also depicted alongside the UFO.

- Orbs are used as messengers by spirits and extraterrestrials to communicate. In this phenomenon, balls of light often make contact. Orbs in the sky can be seen in thousands of online videos within the last 10 years and ongoing. Aboriginal people refer to them as the "Min Min Lights," and are often seen during rituals.

- Crop circles can activate and trigger extraterrestrial contact on Earth. A prime example is the Queensland fire circle, which features images of crafts and spirits as well as fire patterning and triangular shapes.

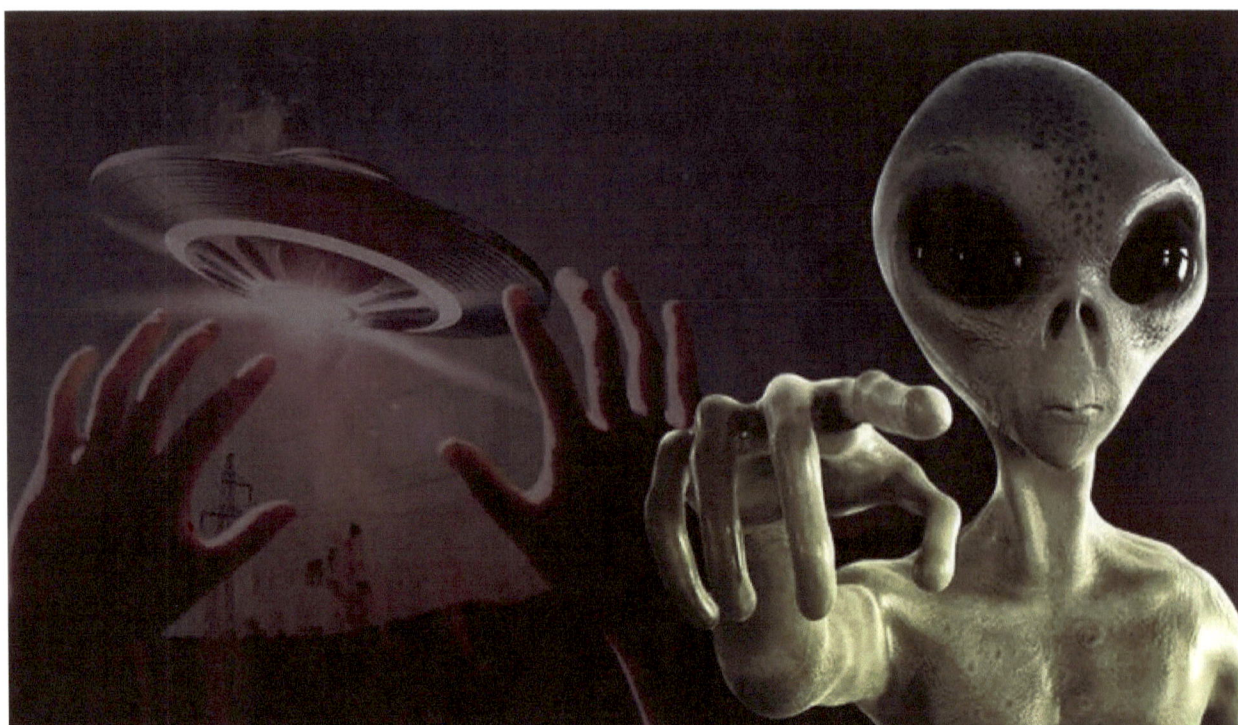

22. **Spiritual Meaning Behind Eye Gazing:** Eyes are known as the windows to the soul, and by looking at someone, you can learn more about them or yourself. It is a subconscious perspective of being aware of someone's light, whether it is positive or negative.

23. **Spiritual Meaning Of Ego Death:** Ego death is an illuminating stage of awakening; it is the loss of self-identity or a rewire in the consciousness that can open up to a lot of positive traits. In ancient and modern philosophy, letting go of the material world of existence was regarded as enlightenment. It is known as breaking the illusion.

24. **Dark Night Of The Soul Meaning:** The "dark night of the soul" is a stage in human development that is brought on by a spiritual crisis that must be overcome in order to gain a perspective on life and figure out one's purpose for existing. This stage is thought to be developmental, and its goal is transformation. During this stage one may question their existence, loss of purpose or meaning, feeling trapped, lack of social support, hopelessness, and so forth.

25. **Spiritual Significance and Afterlife Behind Suicide:** Energy and karmic debt always transfer and manifest into the next life of a being. In the context of suicide, lots of negative vibrations, energy, and karma are tied to it. When a person commits suicide, they will reincarnate into a lesser being or developed form of their previous selves. People who kill themselves experience intense emotions and vibrations in the purgatory state. This purgatory experience is based on their current vibration, energy, and state of frequency they were at before they died. This feeling will feel like hell until they pass into the next stage. In the process, they will also need to ponder how death has affected their loved ones, as they dwell above.

26. **Spiritual Meaning Behind Jinxing:** Jinxing is the practice of conjuring bad fortune and casting a spell. Evil or negative karma might result from emotional wordplay. In fact, occult magic uses the term "jinx" to cast curses or bring about bad luck. Be careful what you wish for and say.

27. Spiritual Meaning Behind DeJaVu: The feeling of recurrence is called Déjà Vu. It's a glitch in the diversions of realms that come back into existence, like when a dream comes back to life. Recollections of past lives, dreams, and messages being delivered to the present are all aspects of DeJaVu.

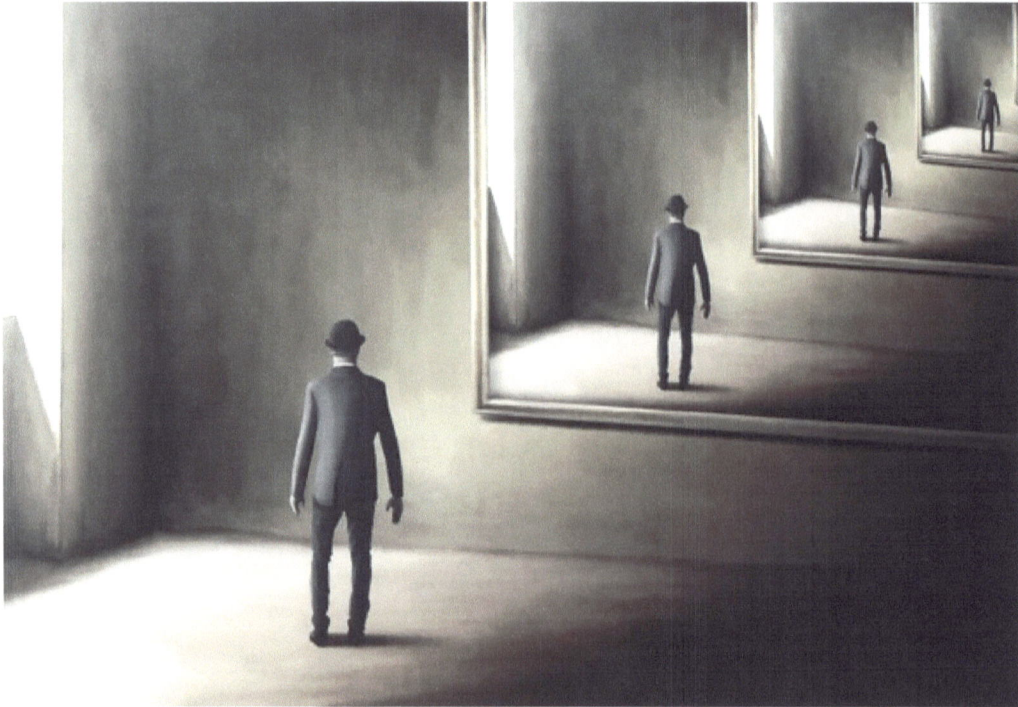

28. Spiritual Meaning Behind Dropping Objects or Breaking Glass: Spirits indicate their presence by silently dropping objects or glasses. They are either leaving or making their presence known. They are described as spirits that wander in the physical world.

29. Spiritual Meaning Behind Wind Blowing/Whistling: When the wind blows or whistles, spirits are said to be entering the environment. They might show up as messengers or as a way of connecting with you and the voices. The wind is a natural force, and communication with spirits is associated with both events.

30. Spiritual Meaning Behind Whistling: Whistling carries the beliefs of summoning spirits and bringing them together. In most cultures, whistling at night brings spirits into the environment. Whistling has the power to foretell events and connect people to favorable or unfavorable outcomes. Numerous folktales state that if you whistle and something answers, it is not a human conversing with you.

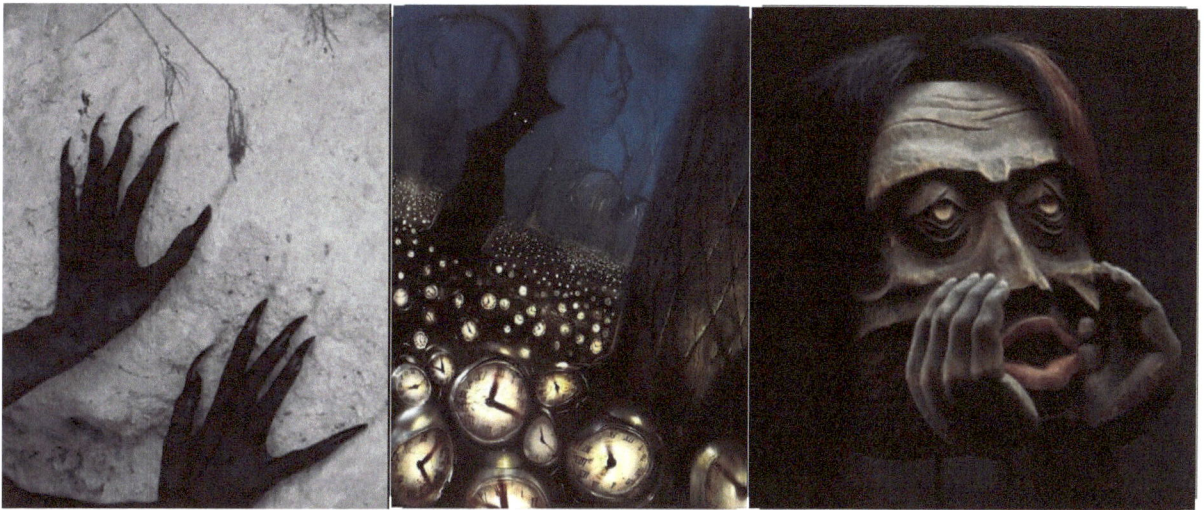

31. Spiritual Meaning Behind Karmic Debt: Everyone experiences karmic debt, which is the repaid karma from a previous life that must be paid back in the current life. You will keep repeating a karmic lesson over and over again if you haven't learned anything from it. Signs of negative relationships, events, luck, and so on, are signs of karmic debt you must go through and overcome, as a result of your actions in the past or in a past life. Karmic debt is repaid through learning lessons and living a moral life.

32. Meaning Behind Spiritual Attacks - Spiritual Warfare

- The psychological aspects are all involved in the daily harassment stemming from hostile conversations, intentions, and pure mind manipulation and tactics to lower your vibration.

- Once you wake up, the spiritual realm understands and knows so. Spirits know everything, they are all knowing, and are intelligent.

- Evil spirits possess other people who have open vessels (unconscious humans/low vibrational beings) in order to work against you and lower your vibration. Family, friends, etc., who are disconnected spiritually and from the source are used to work against light. Oftentimes there are created synchronicities opposed to your own thoughts.

- Spiritual attacks are caused by darkness attracting light; dark energy and entities will always seek to destroy light. The kind of energy that is being sent out will help identify spiritual attacks. Simply remaining resilient and protecting your energy is how to win over them.

- **Biblical Reference - Ephesians 6:12;** "For our struggle is not against flesh and blood, but against the rulers, against the authorities, against the powers of this dark world and against the spiritual forces of evil in the heavenly realms."

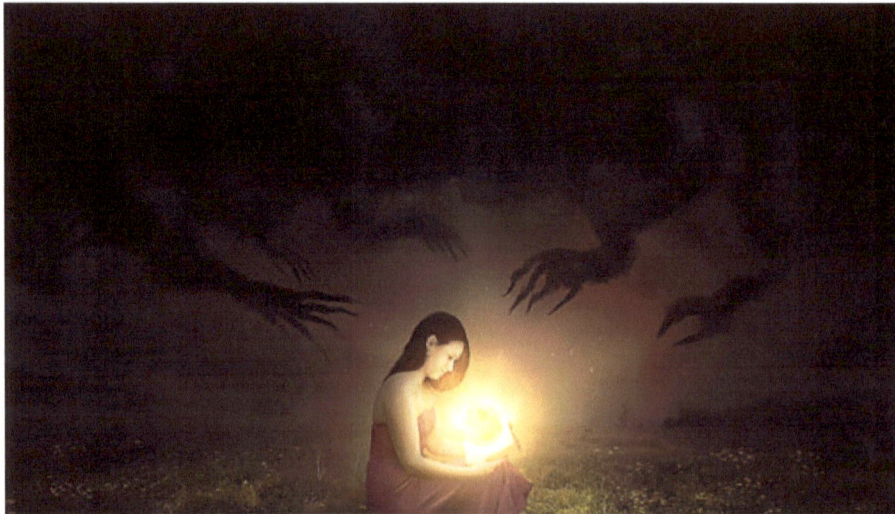

33. **Spiritual Meaning Behind Sudden Cold Hands And Cold Feet:** The spirits of your loved ones (ancestors) have come to check on you. Certain spirits are known to cause our bodies to become chilly whenever they arrive, according to ancient history and traditions.

34. **Spiritual Meaning Behind Crown Chakra**

- The connection to all of the universe's creations is known as the "Crown Chakra." The so-called "god" consciousness. After balancing all of the chakras, it can now be accessed. Through this connection, one's higher self and the universe are interconnected.
- **Symptoms Of Crown Chakra Opening: Physical:** Dizziness, seeing sparks, flashes of light, sensations.
- **Other:** Change of belief, connection to nature, intuition, guided messages and visions.

35. **"Seeing Past The Illusion" - Spiritual Meaning:** The illusion will actually be visible to you, it resembles intense vibratory motions, sparks, static vision (in blue, red, and green), and even eye floaters. This is a reality that is conscious, which is made up of empty space (atoms), generated through every manifested sight.

36. Rejecting Things Subconsciously: Experiences that are kept inside the consciousness can cause things to be rejected for unknown reasons. It is possible to integrate past lives, dreams, and a wide range of events.

37. Spiritual Meaning Behind Sudden Nose Bleeds: You are surrounded by bad energy that is flying or passing by, which is an indication that something is harming you. Nosebleeds are an indication of carelessness.

38. Spiritual Meaning of Butterfly Effect: A butterfly effect happens when a little cause has big consequences. Little adjustments have big effects. Every aspect of reality is interconnected, and the impact of one element ripples across the system.

39. Soul Families: People you meet and instantly connect with without knowing why are called soul families. They are your spiritual family with whom you connect to on a different, deeper, and spiritual level than your physical, third-dimensional family. People who have mindful connections, such as synchronicities, ideas, and the way they think in general, relate to you. According to the Akashic Records, soul families and groups can connect with previous lives and the astral plane (dreams). This reality is full of timelines and different dimensions. Due to the profound harmony experienced, the majority of people intuitively tend to describe this connection as having the same frequency or vibration as each other.

40. Mirror Talk
- Mirror talk is a psychological strategy for improving self-compassion and acceptance.
- Two goals for therapy are to learn to communicate with oneself with compassion and to become conscious of one's inner dialogue.
- You can use a mirror, which is a reflection of you, to change perspectives and bring about changes in your life. A mirror helps you reflect on yourself and transmit messages to your subconscious.

- Keep in mind that the thoughts and feelings you have about yourself are reflected in the mirror. It immediately reveals where you are open and flowing and where you are conflicting.

41. Five Human Senses

- Sight, touch, smell, taste and hearing.
- The five senses of the human body convert vibrational data into electrical signals, which are then transmitted to the brain and, eventually, the entire genetic code. This afterwards decodes into the digital and holographic information that we perceive as the "physical" universe. Simply said, life is just a simulation matrix.

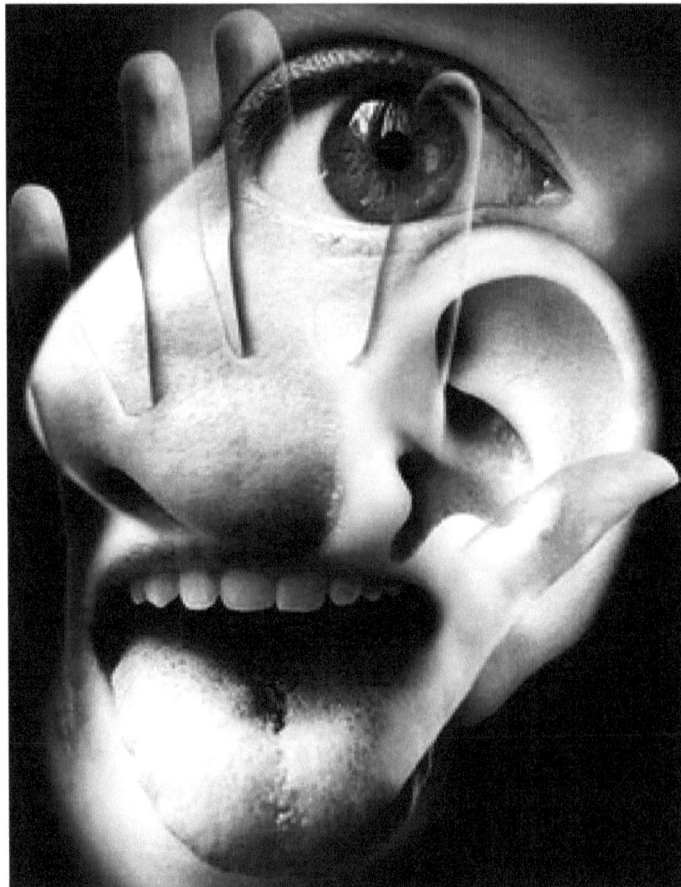

42. **Get Off Your Slumber:** Humans need to get up from their slumber and get off their knees. Millions of people have been killed and millennia of conflict have erupted as a result of religious conflict over who exactly God is and which people have God's approval.

43. Spiritual Attacks in Dreams: Spiritual attacks in dreams are hostile spirits attempting to terrorize the subconscious. For example, frightening nightmares or events that make you feel awful emotions like fear or excessive anxiety. It has been linked with sleep paralysis at times. These experiences imply that certain entities are attempting to exploit or gain from your energy. On rare occasions, it can be associated with encounters with alien life.

44. Spiritual Meaning of Lightning: The clearest example of the electric universe is lightning. A net positive charge flow from the cloud to the Earth causes lightning. Lightning is a manifestation of a heavenly message that honors the chosen. Over the course of history, things have been described in this way.

45. Why To Not Give Your Natal Chart to Certain People or Online

- **Danger Aspect:** Your birth chart contains personal and revealing information. A magician has the option of using the placements and aspects of another person against you. Witches are able to use taglocks in their rituals to cause harm to a person based on anything that relates to them. Such as pictures, birthdays, names, hair or nail clippings, blood and other things. On the other hand, birth charts can be used because they contain specific data that can be linked to a specific thing—typically a person. Hexes are rarely used in this way, but it all depends on who you are and what you do. It is only advised to share with trusted people. You might not want everyone to have access to that kind of private information.

46. More Wisdom The Less You Speak: Your energy and consciousness will increase when you enter the fifth dimension, understand your path in life, and awaken. Due to this change, you won't be able to function on other people's frequency and other people may perceive you differently. Awakening will alter your perspective such that you no longer desire to discuss meaningless (3D topics) things or feel that you no longer can relate to them. This is because you have shifted to a higher frequency.

47. There Are No Coincidences: There are no coincidences. Everything that happened to you, happened for a reason. Whether it's a lesson, karmic debt, or an obstacle. So are the people who came into your lives at certain times and helped you in certain situations. They are the unseen spiritual family taking form in these vessels completing their own tasks.

48. Chakra Signatures: Chakra signatures are handed down through genes. Over time, people may develop specific skills or abilities. Each person has a unique chakra signature, which are the traits they have at birth and have a tendency to emphasize more. For instance, some people could have the throat chakra enhanced and are strong communicators, while others might have the third eye chakra, the capacity to see, feel, and comprehend the energy of others.

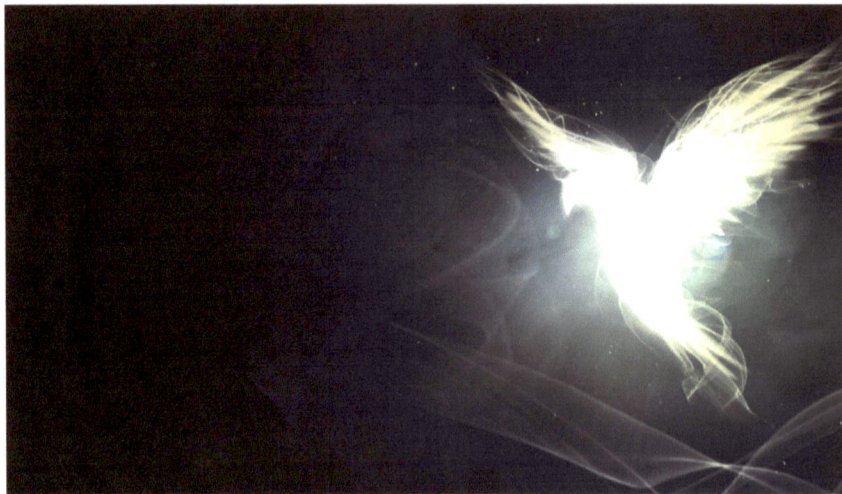

49. Schumann Resonance: Lightning discharges in the ionosphere-surface cavity, create and stimulate global electromagnetic resonances referred to as Schumann resonances. Humans have understood the symbiotic link between the universe and ourselves since the beginning of time. The human aura and our alpha brainwave state synchronize with the aura or heartbeat of the planet.

50. People Staring At You After Awakening
- This can be explained by the auric field that forms when you have a spiritual awakening. You become more attuned to your etheric (light) body, where others can feel and see your presence. You hate it at first, then you question why this is happening, and then you become self-conscious.

- There are many distinct versions of the chosen ones out there, and if you carry this light, remove yourself from the matrix, and become awake, there will be certain individuals who have been programmed to go against you. They look at you strangely and give you the evil eye because they know you have woken up.

- Inception shows a scene in which these two characters actually awaken in the dream (reality), and the deeply programmed people begin to focus on the main characters (hypnosis).

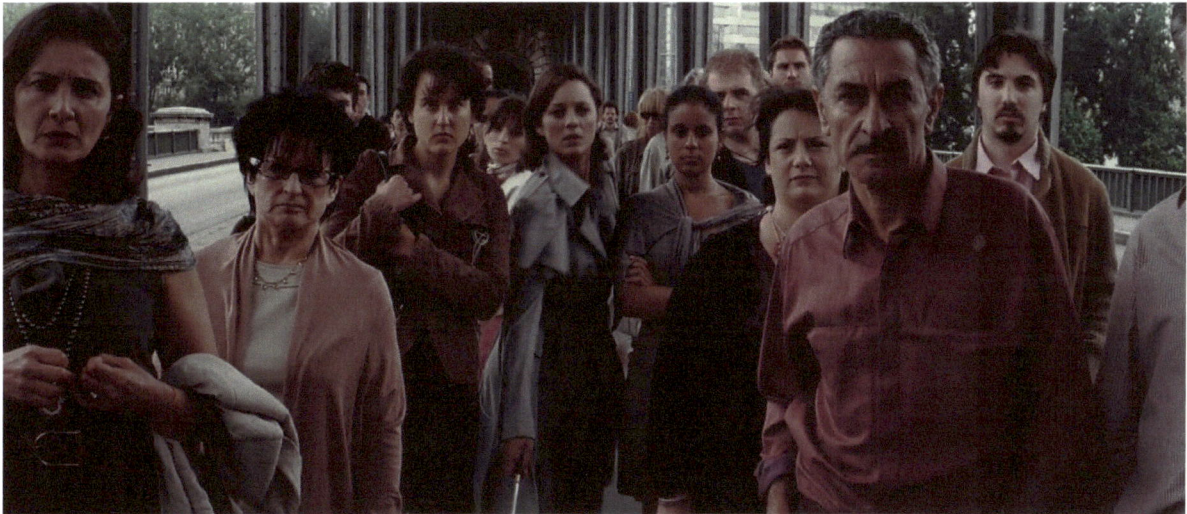

51. Evil Eye: When someone has negative thoughts or intentions toward you, they give you the evil eye, also known as a hostile stare or glare.

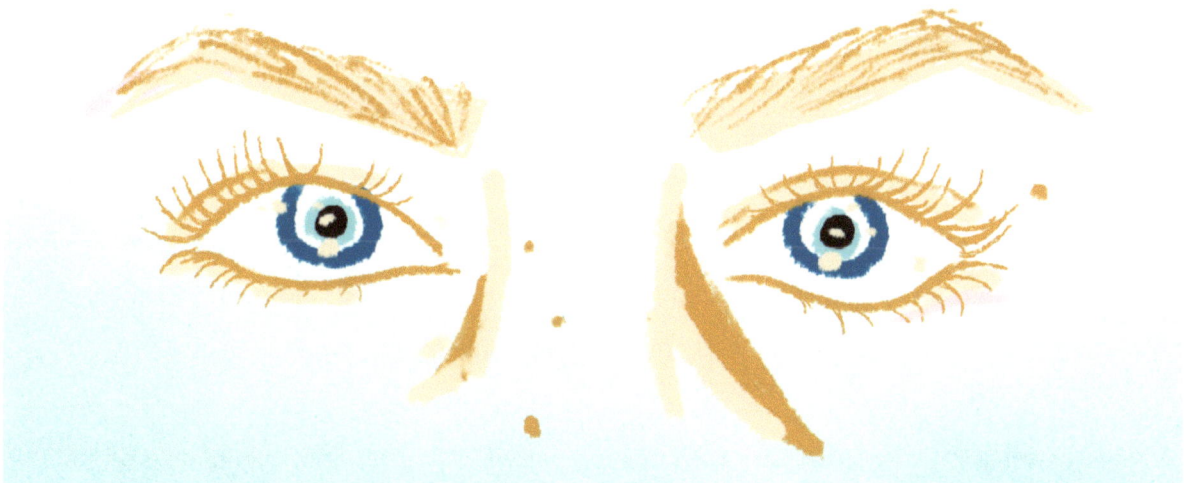

- They are letting you know that they subconsciously discovered who you are. People will actually pay attention to you when you know certain things, which is how energy works. These people can tell when you will enter their space several minutes in advance.

52. **What Are Ghosts:** Ghosts are undead spirits with no awareness of their mortality. They look for hosts who will give them the opportunity to feel more alive. Many other spirits include the docile spirit, the unclean spirit, the lustful spirit, and the spirit of rage. These demons look for hosts who are unaware of their manipulations in order to fulfill their desires.

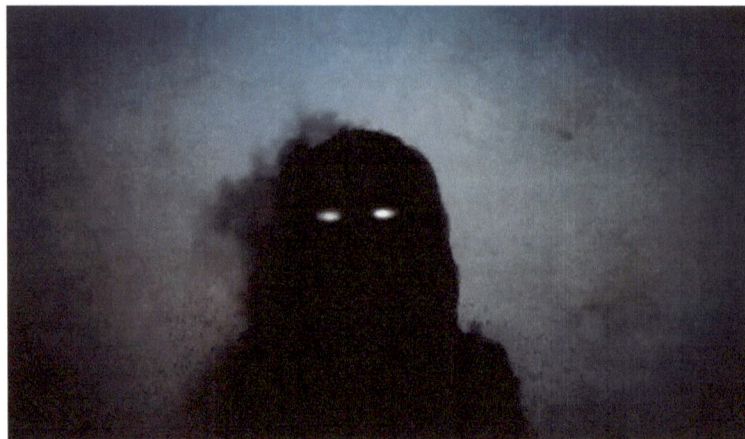

53. **Quantum Discovery:** Quantum physicists found that actual molecules are composed of vortices of energy that are continually turning and vibrating and every one emanating its own special energy signature.

54. **The Matrix:** The universe is made up of particles (such as matter and dark matter) and simulated space. Movement is controlled by algorithms, also known as the laws of physics, physical constants, and quantum unpredictability. This implies that according to The Matrix, humans and their minds are likewise made up of these simulated particles and do not have a physical body that exists outside of the simulation.

55. **Quantum Computer:** The quantum computer is a technology to simulate artificial intelligence. As a result, we beings of the third dimension, must reproduce Time and Space.

56. Mind-Body Function: The basis of the universe is waveform information represented as vibrational resonance. This waveform information structure, which I shall refer to as the "Metaphysical Universe," contains the information fields from where everything manifests. We decode this information into the illusionary "solid" reality that we believe we inhabit every day using the mind-body computer system.

57. Why Time Feels Fast: The Matrix, The Quantum Field, and Universal Consciousness are comparable to quantum computers. On Earth, everyone processes enormous amounts of information through their minds and consciousness to produce a physical warp that speeds up time. This suggests that, collectively, this is the reason we feel like time is passing quickly. Now that both consciousness and world affairs are moving quickly, our awareness and perception need to influence matter on a quantum level.

58. Spiritual Meaning Behind Tattoos: Names, symbols, and logos permeate your energy field with spiritual and vibrational forces. For example, getting a name tattoo of a loved one will enable that person's spirit to stay near to you and carry on living. If a tattoo depicts a particular spirit, divine being, or deity, that profound vibratory energy will attach to it and can be either good or evil. Tattoos have the power to draw spirits and certain energies. When getting tattoos, apply caution because they draw into your blood and can have an impact on your life.

59. What Takes Place Behind Holding Your Seed: Higher levels of consciousness and spiritual enlightenment are attained when you hold your sexual energy, which is the most vital and potent energetic form. Additionally, the energy increase gives one's aura more attraction and gives your manifestations more strength.

60. Spiritual Meaning Behind "Stuck In a Rut": When one does the same actions repeatedly over an extended length of time, they are said to be stuck in a rut. You start to recognise this cycle and start looking for changes through indications and messages you receive from the spirit world.

61. Negative Energies of Animal Meat (Food) - Spiritual: Meat includes negative vibrations, coming from the energy of animals that have been tortured and killed while experiencing emotional distress. As a result, people who eat meat intake the dead animal's negative emotions, toxins, and energy, allowing all negative energy to enter the body. Spiritually, the negative energy that results from eating dead animals can have a wide range of effects, including fatigue, mood swings, and mental unclarity. For this reason, veganism/vegetarianism is incorporated into Buddhism, Hinduism, Jainism, and even Ancient Kemet, four highly spiritual faiths, as it enhances spiritual growth.

62. Curses and Illness - Karmic Debt

Upon the soul's birth into this physical world, the soul chooses what avatar it will inhabit. This includes its conditions, traits, physical features, characteristics, family, and all astrological aspects that are tied to the spirit which gives the avatar an identity for the life to come.

- **(1)** Karmic debt is paid through experiences and life lessons, meaning to learn from mistakes and not make the same selfish or self-destructive errors over and over again. All experiences and activity are attached to the soul and even the auric field, and therefore passed on to the next life stages to come. To put it simply, if one lives a life of utmost chaos, destruction, and a life of low vibrational activity, this in turn, is connected to the soul's karmic debt and must be paid into the next life stage. In most assumed cases, one can experience physical difficulties or harsh environmental conditions that the soul must overcome to advance to the next soul stage.

- **(2)** Those who are born with severe illnesses, restraints, or disabilities, inhabit these bodies with these specific conditions to pay back their karmic debt from what they've done in their previous lives. Subsequently, the soul's journey is to overcome and appreciate life as it is, as it strengthens them with what conditions they are dealing with now.

- **(3)** The soul may also want to experience life with a limited condition to understand how the world is perceived from a limited or unique point of view and make the best of their conditions. Typically in this scenario the person is fully conscious and spiritually awakened that they are aware of their soul and mission on earth.

63. Unspoken Spiritual Side of Schizophrenia

Schizophrenic people have some sort of ESP, (extra-sensory perception) although their brains can be distorted with paranoia and other sorts of cognitive symptoms that can make them seem irrational or crazy. They can see and contact the spiritual realm more closely, such as being able to see auras, spirits, or otherworldly beings. However, they are vulnerable at the same time to hostile spirits, which are often able to manipulate what they are seeing and leech off of their fear and paranoia. Since spirits are all-knowing entities, oftentimes schizophrenic people are contacted by these parasitic spirits and are aware of their conditions, thus they manipulate them often through this field.

- As with all severe medical or cognitive conditions, the soul's purpose is always to be fully aware of it and overcome it. Subsequently, living and overcoming life in a state of peacefulness and equilibrium puts the soul into more advanced positions in the afterlife. The life you are currently living now dictates your life in the future to come.

64. Spiritual Meaning Behind Cats

- Cats have a long history of being revered as sacred and spiritual animals. Cats are renowned for having healing and psychic powers and possessing a sixth sense as well. They possess an extra-sensory perception, enabling them to perceive ghosts, the dead, auras, and different energy fields. They were kept as pets by clairvoyants in the past because they believed they had psychic abilities or could foresee the future. They serve as the spiritual world's protectors and guardian angels. Cats are believed to be able to resist evil energy because of their tremendous astral energy.

- For their own protection, many witches and psychics in medieval Europe kept cats, especially black ones. Cats were the main tool witches employed to protect their sorcerous creations from their own work hazards.

- The belief was so prominent in medieval Europe that people put dried or desiccated cat carcasses (dead cats) inside of walls as protection against spirits. The cats were mostly found deliberately posed in the midst of an attack. Some of these cats were also examined to be alive during these periods. A cat being placed in a wall was thought to be a blood sacrifice in order for the cat to use its psychic abilities to find and fight off evil spirits.

- Cats are often used in sacrificial rituals in many witchcraft manuals to offer their spiritual qualities to pagan gods and to obtain their potent astral energy.

- Cats also possess a powerful healing energy. Researchers from "The Fauna Communications Research Institute" found that every cat in their research produced purr vibrations in the 20–140 Hz range, which are therapeutic for bone growth, healing, pain relief, and swelling reduction.

- Cats have long been connected with mystical phenomena and have even been worshiped as deities. For instance, consider the cat-humanoid Egyptian goddess Bastet, who was revered in ancient Egypt. Egyptians prayed to Bastet to remove disease and guard the household. In order to ward off thieves, they also displayed sculptures of Bastet.

- The term "cats have 9 lives" refers to cats having a higher self-ability, being able to foresee death with their spiritual and natural instincts and avoid them. They also have a unique ability in their flexibility and to maneuver situations that may cause death, which is why they are said to be lucky animals.

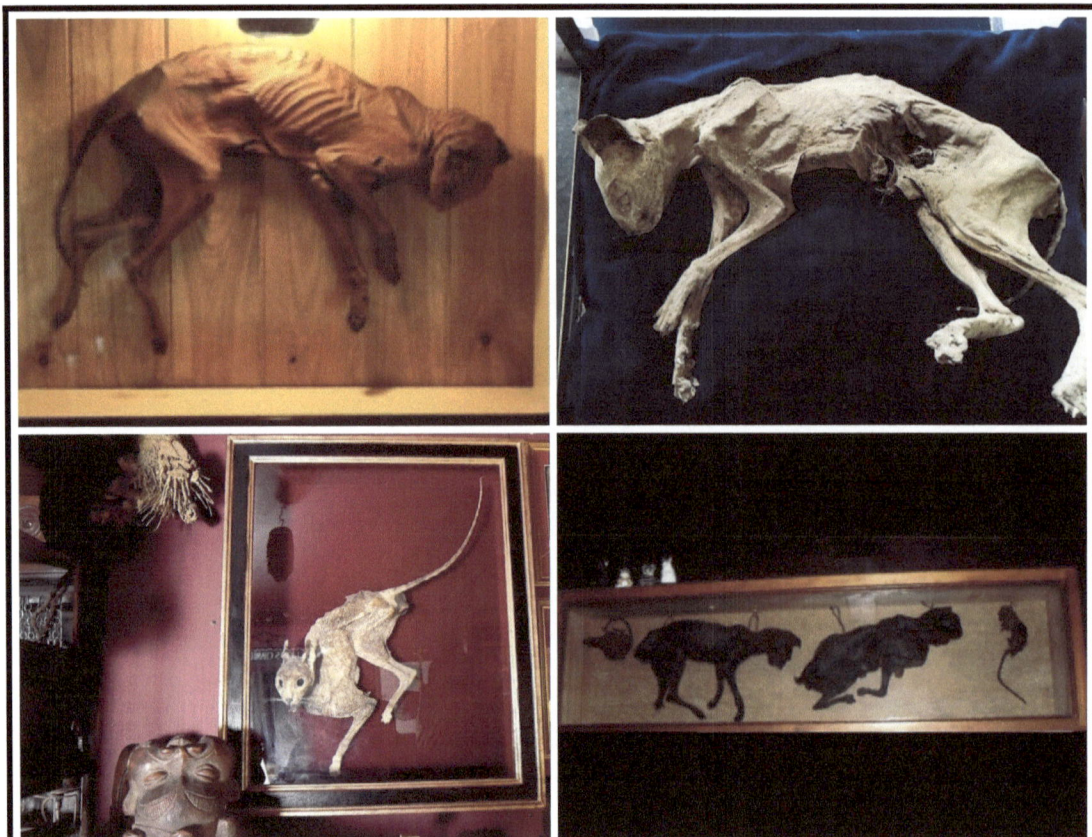

The dried or desiccated carcass of a cat was traditionally placed inside the walls of a newly constructed home in several European cultures to ward off evil spirits or as a good luck charm.

65. Higher Self: The higher self is a person's real self; it is an everlasting, omniscient, conscious, and intelligent being. The evolved being is the part of you that isn't bound by the ego and is one with the universe. However, your lower self is your animalistic side, operating out of the ego with selfish and self-destructive desires.

- Our higher selves are in natural alignment with us, being one step ahead in order to give us directions to certain life situations and choices. The closer we are to ourselves spiritually the more we are tapped into our higher selves and can be guided by divine insight. We become much more rational and guided when we are in alignment with our higher selves. To achieve this, we must operate within the love frequency and find deep connections within our inner selves. Once we can do that, our higher self is able to give us divine insight and directions that are beneficial for us in our life choices.

66. Witch Hour: Spirits that we can physically see with our extra-sensory perception are beings that reside in the 4th dimension. The 4th dimension is a parallel between the 3rd and 5th dimension. During witch hour, between 1 AM and 4 AM is when the physical realm (3D) and the spiritual realm (5D) become the thinnest. These hours are when spirits easily manifest and are active. Calling a spirit's name during these hours is just enough for the room to be filled with spirits.

67. Spiritual Context of Haunted Homes

- People who live very cruel and dark lives, have a spirit and dark energy that remains attached to them, which can include an item, location, or thing. These spirits are often hostile and are limited to either their location or area. Most of the time they are associated with a home. For instance, in families that have been brutally murdered or had a cruel past of abuse, their dark energy and spirit live on. These spirits often hold resentment, sadness, grudges, anger, and such dark energy that they dwell within their attachments to their homes and possessions. These spirits often take their revenge and anger on others.

- This spiritual energy becomes so dark that it can even be felt with an eerie presence. Oftentimes these spirits look to haunt others and possess vessels (humans), in order for their spirit to live on. (this is called body-snatching) In many of these haunted locations, these spirits are often available and contactable.

- This is where you get the spiritual context behind "Haunted Houses" in which we hear many stories, encounters, and also films about this.

- Demons and spirits can attach themselves to clothing, toys, people, etc. They can also mold clothing or objects to the shape of their face.

68. Meaning Behind - Acensionrise

- The meaning behind "Acensionrise" revolves around the word "ACE" meaning 1 (unity), the "ace" counts as the highest even above kings

- Ace = meaning one or unity, "The aim to be one"

- Cension: meaning an assessment. A(cension) a assessment "to be one / united"

- Rise: "evolve" and "grow"

- ACENSIONRISE contains "12" letters which represents perfection, soul mission, entirety, and cosmic order

The Endgame - Blueprint

"Only you can save yourself, no one else, and no outside source can save you, it has to come from within. We can choose to give in to the program and remain slaves, or we can choose to fight it and free our minds. If we all stop participating and giving those people power and control, the game is over. Imagine if millions of people did not go to work one day, buy gas, storm the institutions, the lodges, etc. Imagine if everyone asks to withdraw their money from banks, and we collectively create our own banks, they would collapse and this is the power we have as a people if we come together and unite! Fear, on the other hand, is what is holding us back—concern about the difficulty of making payments on time, which binds us to their illusion and control—and this is the trap they have set for us. They've discovered that convincing a slave that he is free, is the best strategy for keeping him as such…..The elites' greatest concern is that we, the people, will awaken and unite together to reclaim our freedom and power." - **Malik Bade, The Matrix & The Forbidden Knowledge - Extraterrestrial Edition, Page, 69**

Thank you all if you reached all the way up until this point!

Check out the extension of this book "The Matrix & The Forbidden Knowledge - Extraterrestrial Edition" for more additional information. You can find me at @acensionrise on all platforms or at acensionrise@gmail.com.

Full Tables of Content

The series' PDF edition is available on Google Play, with the complete collection of 1204 pages.

Full References (Parts 1, 2, 3, 4, 5)

- The Lost Keys Of Freemasonry, by Manly Palmer Hall, 33°, page 48

- The Secret Doctrine, Helena Petrovna Blavatsky on pages 171, 225, and 255 (Volume II)

- The Secret Doctrine, Helena Petrovna Blavatsky pages 215, 216, 220, 245, 255, 533, (IV)

- Albert Pike, Morals and Dogma, page 102

- The Mysteries Of Magic, Eliphas Levi, page 428

- The Book Of Black Magic, Arthur Edward Waite, 33°, page 244

- The Secret Teaching Of All Ages, Manly Palmer Hall 33° Page CIV

- The Lost Keys Of Freemasonry' Manly Palmer Hall, 33°, page 48

- Albert Pike, Morals and Dogma Page, 321

- The Satanic Rituals, Companion To The Satanic Bible, Anton Szander Lavey

- Albert Pike, Morals and Dogma, Degree I Apprentice

- Support of the United Nations (Lucis Trust). (n.d.). Www.lucistrust.org. Retrieved September 11, 2023, from http://www.lucistrust.org/about_us/support_un
  - Lucis Trust, 1. The World Situation
  - Lucis Trust, 14 XVIII, Page 7 (38)
  - Lucis Trust, "The Esoteric Meaning of Lucifer"

- Education In The New Age, Alice Bailey

- Ruth Montgomery, Threshold to Tomorrow, page 206

- Christopher S Hyatt, Undoing Yourself With Energized Meditation And Other Devices

- The Secret Doctrine, page 245, Helena Blavatsky

- New Age Magazine - "The Official Organ of the Supreme Council 33* - ANCIENT & ACCEPTED SCOTTISH RITE OF FREEMASONRY SOUTHERN JURISDICTION UNITED STATES OF AMERICA - April, 1960 Volume LXVIII, Number, 4,

- Manly P. Hall, 33rd Degree, K.T., The Phoenix: An Illustrated Review of Occultism and Philosophy: (p.176-77)

- R. Swinburne Clymer, The Mysteries of Osiris, 1951, (p. 42)

- Richardson Monitor of Freemasonry, Jabez Richardson

- Scottish Rite Masonry Illustrated - The Complete Ritual - Ancient and Accepted Scottish Rite

- Profusely Illustrated by a Sovereign Grand Commander 33°

- The History of Black Magic, Eliphas Levi

- The Encyclopedia of American Religions, J. Gordon Melton

- Encyclopedia of Freemasonry, page 358, A G Mackey

- The Book of the Law, Aleister Crowley

- The Secret Language, Steve Worrall-Clare

- Morals and Dogma - 29.3 Chapter XXVIII. Knight of the Sun or Prince Adent - Albert Pike

- Richardson's Monitor of Freemasonry on page 142 - Masters Elect of Nine, Jabez Richardson

- Michaël Borremans, Fire from the Sun, Book by Michael Bracewell

- MasonicWorld.com, John Alexander

- Scottish Rite Masonry Illustrated VI The Complete Ritual of The Ancient and Accepted Scottish Rite - By John Blanchard

- Phoenix Masonry. (n.d.). http://www.phoenixmasonty.org/sickles_monitor.htm

- Encyclopedia of Freemasonry, Albert Mackey

- The Secret Doctrine, Helena Blavatsky

- Lucifer: A Theosophical Magazine, March to August 1895, Anne Besant, Helena Blavatsky

- Goodman Magick Symbols, Federick Goodman

- Masonic and Occult Symbols Illustrated, Dr. Cathy Burns, Page 341

- Born in Blood: The Lost Secrets of Freemasonry

- Bertrand Russell, The Impact of Science on Society (1953) pgs. 49-50

- Carl Bernstein: The CIA and the Media

- Office of Dietary Supplements - Fluoride. (2022, April 26). Ods.od.nih.gov. https://ods.od.nih.gov/factsheets/Fluoride-HealthProfessional/

- Connett, P. (2006). Fluoride Action Network | 50 Reasons to Oppose Fluoridation. Fluoridealert.org. https://fluoridealert.org/articles/50-reasons/

- Luke, J. (2001). Fluoride Deposition in the Aged Human Pineal Gland. Caries Research, 35(2), 125–128. https://doi.org/10.1159/000047443

- Dharmaratne, R. W. (2015). Fluoride in drinking water and diet: the causative factor of chronic kidney diseases in the North Central Province of Sri Lanka. Environmental Health and Preventive Medicine, 20(4), 237–242. https://doi.org/10.1007/s12199-015-0464-4

- Council, N. R. (2006). Fluoride in Drinking Water: A Scientific Review of EPA's Standards. In nap.nationalacademies.org.https://nap.nationalacademies.org/catalog/11571/fluoride-in-drinking-water-a-scientific-review-of-epas-standards

- Strunecka, A., & Strunecky, O. (2019). Chronic Fluoride Exposure and the Risk of Autism Spectrum Disorder. International Journal of Environmental Research and Public Health, 16(18), 3431. https://doi.org/10.3390/ijerph16183431

- 50 Reasons to Oppose Fluoridation. (2012, August 7). Fluoride Action Network. https://fluoridealert.org/articles/50-reasons/#:~:text=26)%20 Fluoride%20effects%20 thyroid%20function

- Racial Disparities in Dental Fluorosis. (2012, July 14). Fluoride Action Network. https://fluoridealert.org/studies/dental_fluorosis02/

- Dwardu Cardona, "The Sun Of Night," Kronos Vol. III No. 1 (Fall 1977)

- Lewis M. Greenberg and Warner B. Sizemore,

- "Saturn And Genesis," Kronos Vol. I No. 3 (Fall 1975)

- Immanuel Velikovsky, "On Saturn And The Flood," Kronos Vol. V No. 1 (Fall 1979)

- Tresman, Harold & B. O'Gheoghan (1977), "The 'Primordial Light," SIS, Review Vol II No 2 (December), 35-40

- Lynn E. Rose, "The Lengths of the Year," Pensée Vol. 4 No 3: (Summer 1974) «Immanuel Velikovsky Reconsidered VIII. Referencing: Frederic B. Jueneman, "A Most Exciting Planet," Industrial Research, 15 (July, 1973), p. 11

- Ralph E. Juergens, "The Critics and Stellar Energy," SIS Review Vol IT No 2 (Dec 1977)

114

- Ibid. Velikovsky 1979

- Dwardu Cardona, "Let There be Light," Kronos Vol. III No. 3 (Spring 1978)

- (1980) David Talbott, The Saturn Myth

- Baldwin, Prehistoric Nations

- Manly P. Hall, Secret Teachings of All Ages

- J.S. Ward, Freemasonry and the Ancient Gods

- Eusebius (300AD), Publication Family Magazine: Or Monthly Abstract of General Knowledge, Volume 1

- Bishop Eusebius; Praeparatio Evangelica (I. chs ix-x)

- Gateways To The Otherworld: Gardiner, Philip

- Alfred Dodd, Francis Bacon's Life-Story 1986

Secondary References

- Bilek, J. (2018, February 20). Who Are the Rich, White Men Institutionalizing Transgender Ideology? The Federalist. http://thefederalist.com/2018/02/20/rich-white-men-institutionalizing-transgender-ideology/

- Fraternitas Saturni: Saturn-Gnosis. (n.d.). Pararreligion.ch. Retrieved September 11, 2023, from http://pararreligion.ch/fs3.htm

- montalk. (n.d.). Spiritless Humans | Transcending the Matrix Control System. Montalk.net. Retrieved September 11, 2023, from http://montalk.net/matrix/157/spiritless-humans

- Jay Myers Documentary - MK Ultra Mind Control (Documentary)

- Jay Myers Documentary - Ghislaine Maxwell

www.ingramcontent.com/pod-product-compliance
Lightning Source LLC
Chambersburg PA
CBHW041239020426

42333CB00002B/21